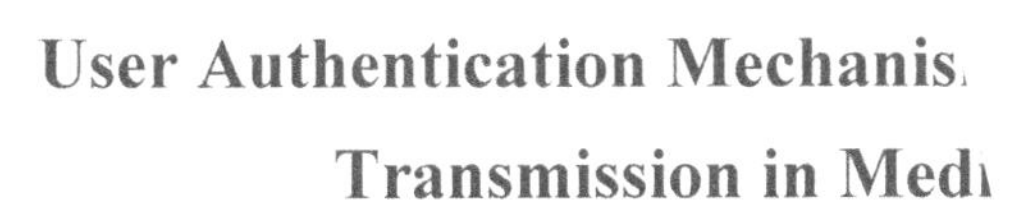

User Authentication Mechanis
Transmission in Med

Jyotheeswari P

TABLE OF CONTENTS

LIST OF TABLES

LIST OF FIGURES

LIST OF SYMBOLS AND ABBREVIATIONS

ABE	-	Attribute-Based Encryption
AKE	-	Authenticated Key Exchange
AMQP	-	Advanced Message Queuing Protocol
COAP	-	Constrained Application Protocol
DDoS	-	Distributed Denial Of Service
DoS	-	Denial of Service
ECC	-	Elliptic Curve Cryptography
IoT	-	Internet of Things
KDF	-	Key Derivation Function
M- IOT	-	Medical Internet of Things
MITM	-	Man in The Middle Attack
M2H	-	Machine-to-Human
M2M	-	Machine-to-Machine
MQTT	-	Message Queuing Telemetry Transport
PAKE	-	Password Authenticated Key Exchange
PIA	-	Privacy Impact Assessment
PKES	-	Passive Key level Entry and Start system
RFID	-	Radio Frequency Identification
SSL	-	Secure Socket Layer
WSNs	-	Wireless Sensor Networks
XMPP	-	Extensible Messaging and Presence Protocol

CHAPTER 1

INTRODUCTION

1.1 Internet of Things

The Internet of Things (IoT) contains sensors, microcontrollers, network software, and actuators embedded in things (i.e. physical objects). IoT comprises of a vast number of smart devices rather than gadgets connected through the internet, such as smartphones, refrigerators, automobiles, industrial and health care units. Based on the opinion of Ericsson, by the end of 2022, more than 29 million devices will be connected through the IoT. The primary aim of the IoT is to connect the objects using the inter-routing protocol and software. These smart devices exchange the data with the server or connected nodes. The applications of IoT in different fields are increasing rapidly. For instance, the IoT can be used to find locations, track patients' heart rate, and find the movement in the vehicles and products.

IoT provides additional advantages to the technologies that serve urban areas where there is scope in health care. IoT has the additional benefit to serve in health care like patient monitoring at home. IoT contains a huge volume of heterogeneous devices and is connected with the internet. The web technologies which support IoT are XML, HTML, and JSON. A major advantage of using web technologies is that they are supported by devices integrated with the existing infrastructure.

The IoT could be characterized as a pervasive and ubiquitous network which enables monitoring and control of the physical environment by collecting, processing, and analyzing the data generated by sensors or smart objects.

Additionally, it consolidates Machine-to-Human correspondence (M2H), Radio Frequency Identification (RFID), Location-Based Services (LBS), Lab-on-a-Chip (LOC) sensors, Augmented Reality (AR), apply self-sufficiency and vehicle telematics. Countless advances are the eventual outcome of changes in military and present-day stock system applications; their typical component is to join introduced substantial articles with correspondence understanding, running data over a mix of wired and remote frameworks. In a broader association, the configuration fuses the Internet of Things notwithstanding business building bits of learning acquired from the information transmitted by these gathered "keen items". The middle end degree of this paper is on the security point of view (generally connected with confirmation) of the Internet of Things.

The ability of embedded and distributed intelligence in the network is a core architectural part of the IoT for three fundamental reasons:

- Data Collection: Centralized data gathering and organization do not give the versatility required by the internet. Case in point, managing a couple of million sensors and actuators in a Smart Grid framework is inconceivable using a joined technique.

- Network Resource Preservation: Because framework exchange pace may be uncommon, gathering natural data from a vital issue in the framework unavoidably prompts using a considerable measure as far as possible.

- Closed Loop Functioning: For some use cases, the IoT requires diminished reaction times. For instance, sending an alert through various hops from a sensor to a fused system (which runs examination) before sending a solicitation to an actuator would include unacceptable deferrals.

This passed-on knowledge capacity is known as Fog Computing, a building especially expected to process data and events from IoT gadgets closer to the source than a focal server farm (generally called "Cloud"). In summation, Fog Computing is an advancement of the cloud perspective. It resembles circulated registering, close towards the earths surface. The Fog Computing outline enlarges the cloud stretched out physically to the universe of things.
Service Management Systems (SMS) generally called Systems of Network Management, Management Systems, or back end structures constitute the brainy part inside an IoT plan. SMS interfaces with sharp databases consisting of contract information, insightful capital information, information related to course of action, and even for delivering specific data. Such SMS, in addition, reinforces picture affirmation developments to perceive objects, people, structures, spots, logos, and the rest of them possess and offer quality to buyers and endeavors. PDAs and tablets containing cameras extend such developments from general mechanical type applications to broader buyers and

endeavor applications. The data supported by such kinds of relevant structures fecilitate further development.
When in doubt, an important interference of the standard model is its particular course of action and challenges. Some security challenges and examinations in laying out and fabricating IoT gadgets or structures are:

- Typically little efficient devices serve for all intents and purposes but may not provide physical security.

- Computing stages, constrained in memory and register resources, may not support unpredictable and propelling security estimations as a result of the facts that go with components: Limited security figure limits, encryption figures need higher planning power and Low CPU cycles versus reasonable encryption.

- Designed to work in a self-governing way in the field with no fortification system (if the fundamental affiliation is lost).

- Mostly presented before framework openness which extends all things considered on-stacking uptime.

- Requires secure remote organization in the midst of and in the wake of onboarding.

- Scalability and organization of billions of substances in the IoT natural framework.

- Identification of endpoints versatility like an individual unit. To cite a gadget: Home Smart Meter, or Group.e.g., All lights in a room/home, Scalability troubles of individual versus gathering. At times the range might be more imperative than the Individual Identifier (ID).

- Management of Multi-Party Networks for occurrence. E.g: Smart Traffic Lights, a situation where there can be a couple of contributed people, for instance, Emergency Services (User), Municipality (proprietor), Manufacturer (Vendor), Crypto Resilience i.e. Embedded devices may outlive figuring life time. For example,

Smart meters could last recent years and crypto estimations have a limited life-time before they are broken (Scarpato et al., 2014).

- Physical Protection i.e., theft of mobile contraptions or moving away of fixed devices.

- Tamper detection techniques and layout: It may always be on: High Poll rate, highly imperative, quicker revelation, Periodic Poll: essential to a small extent, slower distinguishing proof and now and again Push: It is for minimum essential type, no acknowledgment will be received.

The gadgets and the control stage on which information might be expanded and shared could have diverse possession, arrangement, administrative, and network areas. Thus, gadgets are expected to possess equivalent and open accessibility to various information purchasers and controllers simultaneously, while holding security and selectiveness of information where it is required between those shoppers. Data accessibility, while giving information disconnection between normal clients is rudimentary. There is a need to set up proper character controls as well as fabricate trust connections among substances for sharing the correct data.
It looks contending that the security of complex type prerequisites are to be sent on a stage with possibly restricted assets like:

(i) Authentication of different systems safely.

(ii) Ensuring that information is accessible to numerous gatherers,

(iii) Manage the dispute in information access,

(iv) Managing security concerns among various buyers,

(v) Providing solid verification and information insurance (honesty and secrecy) that are not effectively bargained,

(vi) Maintaining accessibility of the information or administration and

(vii) Allowing the advancement despite obscure dangers.

Such problems are of specific significance in the IoT, as secured accessibility of information is of vital significance. To cite an instance, a basic mechanical procedure might depend upon precise as well as approximate temperature estimation. On the off chance that there is an endpoint experience, a Denial of Service (DoS) assault, the procedure gathering operator should be one means or another be made mindful. On such an occasion, the framework ought to be capable of taking fitting activities progressively. Sourcing information from an optional association or postponement of data transmission can be referred as an example. It should likewise have the capacity to recognize. Loss-of-information as there can be an ongoing DoS assault leading to the gadget in the plant being lost because of a calamitous occasion. This may be fulfilled by utilizing learning machine methods (for instance, contrasting an ordinary operational state with an assault state already learned).

Rahmani and Amir (2018) proposed that IoT is a multi-layered architecture in both theoretical and practical ways. For instance, sensor devices in the IoT gather the data of the patients and forward it to the gateways. These sensors and gateways are nearer to each other. Here , the router is the gateway placed in the room of the patient. These gateways forward the information to the cloud for storage and further analytics. It was interesting for them to know about the communication that took place between the IoT devices. CISCO studied IoT architecture with seven layers. The goal of this architecture is to define and describe the functionality of IoT applications. The first layer in the architecture is associated with edge nodes such as smart readers, sensors, and RFID tags. The second layer is associated with communication, where the components are communicating within or between the layers. The third layer is edge computing where simple communication takes place to reduce the computational load and for a fast response. The fourth layer is called data accumulation where it transforms the motion data into data at rest. To cite an instance, the stored data are in the database. The fifth layer is related to the data abstraction where the data is processed for further use with modesty and efficiency. The sixth layer is associated with applications. This layer provides the interpretation of the information. The final layer is composed of users and data centers, where the user utilizes the applications and the associated data in the data centers.

Ouaddah et al., (2017) proposed the three layers of architecture for simplifying the CISCO model. First, the sensor nodes, data communication, and edge computing are grouped to form the sensor side layer. Next, the data communication and abstraction layers are grouped into cloud-side layers. Finally, the applications, users, and data cen-

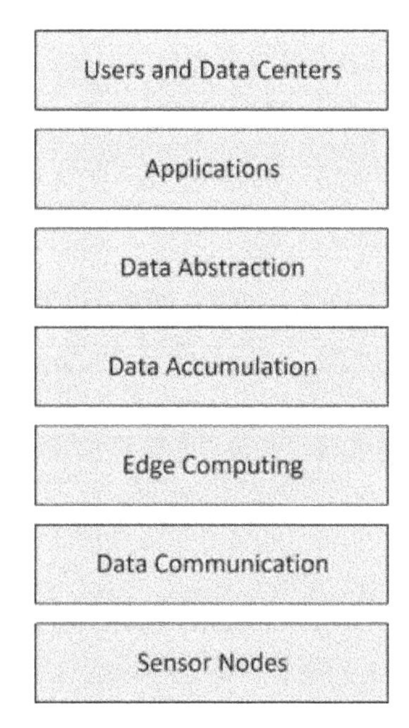

Fig. 1.1 CISCO IoT Reference Architecture(CISCO,2014)

ter layers are grouped into the user-side layer.

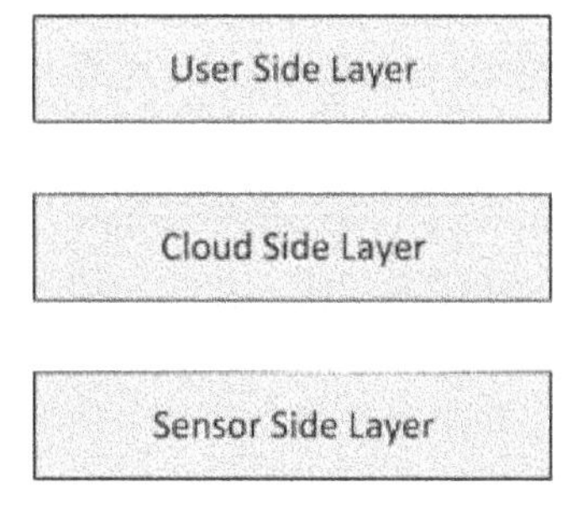

Fig. 1.2 IoT Reference Architecture (Ouaddah et al., 2017)

In some of the research works, the architecture of IoT in health care composed of sensor nodes, IoT gateways, back-end services, and applications. As such, the essential parts of the health care IoT architecture are given as follows:

a) Sensor Nodes: The sensor nodes in the health care IoT are responsible for gathering the sensed data and forwarding data to the gateway. The sensor nodes support different types of wireless communications to communicate with IoT devices.

b) IoT Gateway: This device is more crucial in the IoT architecture, which connected the sensor nodes with remote back-end services with the help of IPV4 or IPV6 protocols. IoT gateway provides temporary storage, converts the protocols, and manages the devices. The IoT gateway interconnects the local devices to the remote devices.

c) Back-end services: The back-end services are offered by the third party or by self-development. The back-end services provide storage services to store the sensor data, analytical services to make the decisions. These back-end services also offer security and help to integrate different tools to analyze the sensor data.

d) Applications: These applications are installed in the users smartphone or desktop to monitor the IoT services.

1.2 Communication Patterns of IoT

The IoT communication pattern is studied based on the layers. Tschofenig et al., (2015) proposed the four IoT communication patterns: Object-to-Object communication, Object-to-Cloud communication, Object-to-Gateway communication, and data sharing with servers.

a) Object-to-Object Communication:
Two or more objects are communicated by connecting directly with each other. This type of communication normally takes place in applications with small size packets and low bandwidth to communicate between the objects. This type of communication has built-in security and trusted principles. The major challenge faced by Object-to-Object Communication is interoperability (Baker et al., 2017).

b) Object-to-Cloud Communication:
In Object-to-Cloud communication, the nodes at the network end collect the data and forward it to the cloud servers. This type of communication follows the IP- based approach like Wi-Fi or Ethernet.

c) Object-to-Gateway Communication:
In Object-to-Gateway communication, the nodes at the end of the network are connected to the gateway. This gateway acts as a middle layer between the object and the cloud. For instance, smartphones, routers, hubs, and controllers acts as gateways (Kinkelin Holger et al., 2018).

1.3 Health care IoT

Researchers have contributed with many approaches to health care IoT. The IoT is integrated with different technologies to develop new health care mechanisms like e- health, medical IoT, smart home, health care, and smart health (Bennett et al., 2017; Scarpato Noemi et al., 2017; Kang et al., 2018). The Health care IoT provides services for health care requirements. For instance, IoT could be used to monitor the patients at home and provide health care without the need to visit the hospital. The medical IoT is also used in hospitals, cities, and doctors offices (Ericsson, 2018). The IoT devices used in health care are heart rate sensors, wearable sensors, diabetes sensors, oxygen saturation sensors, and many more. Alpr Gergely et al., (2016) suggest the usage of IoT in many applications of health care areas like monitoring chronic diseases and disabilities.

Not with standing the security and privacy, risks grew proportionally. Huge data quantity are at times securely processed, transmitted as well as stored. The disruption of communication channels could prevent patients from receiving health care in an emergency. Data breaches on patients medical records could cause societal pressure, embarrassment, and discrimination. Systems could be potentially misused to the patients detriment. Privacy infringements could be caused by, e.g., purpose misuse, vague purpose specification, lack of patients consent, and privacy policies. Furthermore, in most countries, there is no legal framework regulating privacy and protection of personal data.

The main reasons for using the Health care IoT are as follows:

- Decreased cost inpatient treatment
- Improved patient care
- Remote monitoring
- Extended health care services to rural areas
- Good access to doctors for immediate care
- Doctors can treat a large number of patients

Despite having the different advantages of health care IoT, security and privacy are the major two challenges IoT. Security is one of the issues that makes an obstacle to the progress of IoT in different fields. The traditional security mechanism cannot be applied to the IoT. It is due to the fact that the nodes in the IoT have limited computation capacity and battery power. The public key encryption cannot be applied to the IoT environment. Therefore, IoT devices require saleable solutions to provide security by using limited computation capacity. Researchers (AlabaFadele et al., 2017; Kouicem et al., 2018; Alphand et al., 2018; Antonio et al., 2010) have proposed several security algorithms, tools, frameworks, procedures, and certificates to provide security to the IoT. They have developed lightweight encryption algorithms to provide security to the IoT. But, what they lack is proper implementation procedure. As a result, security and privacy are the major issues in the IoT.

Song et al., (2003) proposed searchable-based encryption for text search in the encrypted data. This work gained more attention from researchers and encouraged research in the keyword search issues on the ciphertext. Goh et al., (2003) proposed attribute-based encryption. This method contains both ciphertext and secret keys which are associated with attributes set. The retrieving of a message is possible from ciphertext if the users key is matched with the ciphertext attributes.

Bettencourt (2017) mentioned that the RFID reader can scan customers RFID tags unnoticed by them. An unauthorized intruder can do accessing of customers information. Such an act can be easily done while transmitting information from the local server towards the remote server (Raju and Saritha, 2016). In IoT, mostly the network that communicates utilizes small sensors by count. Apart from that, algorithms with lightweight encryptions are utilized for encrypting the data (Medaglia and Serbanati, 2009). Groce et al., (2010) proposed the security protocol with higher proven security in the generalized model. It does not suit handling the medical-IoT applications. Forsstrm et al., (2010) surveyed on security issues of IoT concerning different heterogeneous networks and they managed to develop the distributed verification method for user authentication. However, this method is not suitable to deal with real-time dynamic data.

1.3.1 Security and Privacy for Health care

High-quality health care requires individuals to share their personal health information with health care professionals (Kouicem et al., 2018). Furthermore, the information should be complete and accurate. If patients cannot trust that their information will be safe, they will be reluctant to share it (or even to use the service). If health professionals cannot trust the organization to keep records secured, they will not store complete information there. In both cases, this leads to inferior health care. It is therefore paramount that privacy and security concerns are addressed during the design and development of any health information system.

For the sake of clarity, this part of the background is organized into four macro topics:

(1) general concerns on security and privacy;

(2) security mechanisms;

(3) Privacy Impact Assessment (PIA);

(4) data obfuscation and anonymization.

That is, moving from the general to the specific concepts.

Essentially, M- IoT inherits problems from mobile computing and wireless networks. The communication channels are more vulnerable due to their wireless characteristics (e.g., network eavesdropping and spoofing) and mobile devices have a more constrained amount of processing power and memory (i.e., need for lightweight cryptography). Devices can be shared among users, and they are more vulnerable to theft, loss, and damage, which may result in data breaches, data loss, and privacy infringements.
You et al., (2011) proposed several security and privacy recommendations for m-health developers, from a more technical perspective. These recommendations are made based on a preliminary survey, resulting in eight general recommendations listed below:

1. Access control: Use of patient-centered access control mechanisms (e.g., role-based access control), in which users shall be enabled for permitting and also even to refuse to access their information at whichever instant they need to do so.

2. Authentication: Clients should be able to authenticate using a unique ID as well as a password (or multi-factor authentication). Passwords should be kept in secrecy and it shall attain an apt security level.

3. Confidentiality: Utilizing mechanisms for encrypting (e.g., AES) with proper parameter configurations (i.e., size of a key).

4. Integrity: Use of message authentication codes and digital signatures, Inform patients the privacy policy is presented to clients before data collection- that is, informing that clients about their rights and clarifiying the reason for data collection and also the reason for doing the process with them.

5. Data transfer: Use secure communication channels (e.g., TLS, VPNs) while transferring data among entities. Notify the user regarding the transferring of data.

6. Data retention: Inform clients about the policy regarding data retention. The data shall be kept during the required period alone for a prior specified reason. A client must be able to check deletion of data after it is done.

7. Body Area Network communication: Use mechanisms of security to authenticate and distribute keys between sensors and smartphones. Also, establish secure communication channels among the devices.

8. Breach notification: In the case of data breaches, the competent authorities and users should be notified. The entity concerned must help clients related to relieving the consequences as well as restoring possibly occurred damages.

Overall, the recommendations help developers to have a glimpse of privacy and security issues in m-health. However, they are incomplete if compared to the existing legislation on privacy and data protection, and thus, have limited practical use. For example, in the case of the European Union (EU), the General Data Protection Regulation (GDPR) Forsstrm et al., (2012) is the upcoming regulation for personal data privacy and protection, replacing the EU Data Protection Directive 95/46/EC (Rahmani et al., 2018).

However, many countries (i.e., separate legal jurisdictions) do not have specific legislation for data privacy (Gronbaek, 2008). This does not imply a legal void in the area, but privacy rights might stem from the constitution or consumer rights; and in the case of health care, from medical codes of conduct, and so on. Thus, from a legal perspective, some publications help to bridge this gap between privacy and m-health technologies. For example, Yang et al., (2012) present a list of five guiding principles for mobile privacy in the context of developing countries (that map to principles of the GDPR):

Principle 1: Address Surveillance Risks- Projects should take steps to ensure that user data is secured from third-party surveillance, e.g., user discriminatory profiling can be made by mobile operators and the government.

Principle 2: Limit Data Collection and Use -Projects should limit data collection to what is absolutely necessary for the projects goal, e.g., by employing access control, data retention policy, and not collecting unnecessary data.

Principle 3: Promote and Facilitate Transparency-Projects should be transparent about what data is collected, how it is shared, and how it might be used in the future e.g., user notifications, data transfer policies, audit trails of others that also have access to the data.

Principle 4: Incorporate User Feedback - Projects should give users the ability to access, amend and/or delete their data, e.g., create user interfaces, create communication channels to receive feedback from users.

Principle 5: Assume Responsibility - Projects should assume accountability for potential risks and harms incurred via their projects and platforms, e.g., perform risk assessment, plan an incident response and notify data breaches.

The content of the recommendations (You et al., 2011) and the guiding principles (Istepanian, 2011) offer a good starting point for developers and project leaders. However, in practice, security and privacy analysis should be done case-by-case, given the complexity, multiplicity of actors, jurisdictions, and highly culture-specific dimensions of privacy (Castillejo et al., 2013).

1.3.2 Security Mechanisms for M-IoT

Some fundamental cryptographic mechanisms and protocols are used in research. In brief, a Key Management Mechanism (KMM) is used to provide Authentication and Key Exchange (AKE) between parties (users mobile and application server). Authentication protocols and key derivation schemes for MDCSs usually rely on symmetric cryptography, using password authentication. These protocols should also give support for online and offline user authentication. Other mechanisms should cope with the confidentiality of stored and in-transit data, using encryption schemes for secure storage and transmission. As a result, the security background here is presented as the building blocks of solutions.

1.3.3 Authentication and Key Derivation

Authentication of users remains a challenging and crucial aspect of new computer security. The mechanisms for authenticating can indeed be pivoted on a combination of factors i.e., biometrics (what the user is), security tokens (what the user has), or passwords (what the user knows) the widely existing strategy yet lies in secret passwords (Istepanian et al., 2011). This happens because password-based authentication is the most well-known, simple, cost-effective, and efficient method of maintaining a shared secret between a human being and a computer system. Furthermore, the advantages of using passwords tend to mitigate the drawbacks, i.e., issues related to selecting strong but easily remembered passwords. Hence, it is expected that one might see passwords being in use for a while in the near future (by themselves or as part of multi-factor authentication schemes (Ruiz et al., 2009)).

The password-based systems normally utilize Key Derivation Functions (KDFs) algorithms of cryptography type that allow the function of generating a string of bits of pseudo-random type from the very password. In a typical way, the KDFs output is utilized in one of the two ways: one is local storing as a token form for verifications of the password in the near future, ard the other, it might be utilized with secrecy as the Secure and Privacy-aware Data Collection and Processing in Mobile Health Systems key to doing encrypting and/or authenticating of data. Whatever be the case, these solutions internally utilize a one-way function (e.g., hash), such that recovery of the password from the KDFs output turns out to be computationally infeasible (Trnka et al., 2018). Nonetheless, attackers might yet utilize dictionary attacks and test varying password combinations until a matching one is identified (i.e., brute force). KDFs normally rely on a couple of rudimentary strategies to prevent these brute-force attacks. The first one is raising the costs involved of each guessed password in terms of computational resources, like time to process and/or usage of memory. The second one is for taking as input apart from the user-memorable password, random bits in a sequence called salt. The mentioned random variable prevents many attacks pivoted on tables of prior-built common passwords, i.e., it forces the attacker to create a fresh table from the beginning for each different salt. The mentioned salt may be looked upon as an index into a large key set possible, arrived from the password that does not require clients' memorization, or maintained in secrecy.

1.3.4 Password-based Remote Authentication and Key Exchange

In principle, KDFs could be used for data delivery. If the local and remote systems share the same password, they could exchange data by revealing the salt employed for generating the key that protects such data. However, since this would allow attackers to use the same salt in an offline dictionary attack, KDFs are usually employed only for local data storage, establishing a secure channel between the human user and the local system.

Delivering data for remote locations is generally found to utilize protocols of Password Authenticated Key Exchange (PAKE). These methods allow two or even more parties who can share a password for authenticating one another. It creates a secure channel for protecting communication. To ensure it as a secured one, solutions of PAKE must ensure that a party that is not authorized (that is fully controlling the channel used for communicating while it doesnt discern the password) will be able to know the key results. It can not do guess work of the password utilizing even offline attacks of brute force.

The Secure Remote Password (SRP) project group Dohr et al., (2010) describes the following attacker model for PAKE protocols:

(a) Attackers have complete knowledge of the protocol.

(b) Attackers have access to a large dictionary of commonly used passwords.

(c) Attackers can eavesdrop on all communications between client and server.

(d) Attackers can intercept, modify, and forge arbitrary messages between client and server; and

(e) A mutually trusted third party is not available.

Looking briefly into the history of PAKE protocols, the Encrypted Key Exchange (EKE) (Kinkelin Holger et al., 2018) is probably the first successful proposal. Although several of the published methods are flawed, the surviving and enhanced forms of EKE have effectively amplified the security of using passwords to establish shared keys for confidential communication and authentication. Other provably- secure PAKE include the schemes described in Scarpato, Noemi et al., (2017) (which uses the standard model) and in Baker et al., (2017) (which uses the random oracle model). These groups of EKE-inspired proposals are commonly referred to as the EKE family of protocols.

1.3.5 Forward Secrecy Property

The security of computer systems relies upon the fact that those who attack cannot access a secret that underlies it (Imadali et al., 2012). In practice, however, achieving this condition can be challenging. As a result, most strategies are used to minimize exposing the secret keys, increase the prices, or affect the systems usability (e.g., multi-factor authentication mechanisms). Therefore, one must assume that a striving intruder might successfully expose the secrets of the system (especially when using PAKE), and we should explicitly deal with such events and elaborate strategies to minimize potential damages.

One approach is to use (password-based) protocols that have the so-called forward secrecy also called perfect forward security property (Trnka et al., 2018). For the methods of AKE, the property mentioned may be stated in the following manner: in case the long-term secret information e.g., the password is disclosed to an attacker, such facts cannot help obtain ephemeral keys (i.e., session keys derived from the long-term secret) from earlier communicated transactions, protecting the entire exchange of information done earlier (Shahamabadi et al., 2013). That is, consider a situation where the parties that participate in the protocol share a long-term secret S. Then do running of the protocol r times before S is compromised by the one who attacks. Now the attacker is not able to find the ephemeral keys set K, Kr created before such disclosure of S. The keys created subsequently, that is Kr + i where ($i > 0$) produced utilizing that S only could be compromised by the mentioned attacker.

This principle forms the integrating part of several security solutions in recent times, inclusive of digital signatures, pseudo-random generators and public-key encryption (Istepanian, 2011). Generally, it is utilized to secure data channels for limited/temporal interaction (i.e., keys expire and should change). Moreover, there is a possibility for utilizing the principle of forwarding secrecy to secure storing of data, as it avoids encrypting of data in huge amounts with a single secret key (e.g., as done in Open PGPs (KangMinhee et al., 2018) and e-mail encryption (Istepanian et al., 2004). Whatever the case, the main shortcoming in utilizing forward secrecy is that the strategy causes additional operations. It leads to a technique of complex key evolving or management.

1.3.6 Secure Data Storage

At the time that user and server agree on a common shared key (e.g., the ephemeral keys aforementioned) by employing a PAKE protocol, this key might be utilized for protecting the stored data in the mobile phone. This secure storage mechanism should encrypt all the sensitive information that will reside in the mobile storage (e.g., configuration files, users data) and the in-transit data that is temporarily stored and sent to the server. Hence, encryption assures data confidentiality letting only authorized parties read data. This mechanism will use sufficiently lightweight encryption algorithms owing to the devices limited processing and memory capacity. However, as pointed out, encryption carries the risk of making data unavailable due to data transformation, or if anything goes wrong with the key management process (Mosa et al., 2012). In other words, developers should be aware that the key management adds complexity at least on the server-side as it is necessary to store partial values to rebuild users keys to decrypt and consolidate the data received.

1.3.7 Privacy Impact Assessment

Privacy is not only for personal data protection, as already mentioned, but it also has a broader dimension and is more complex in nature than security. For someone to understand privacy, it is crucial to comprehend its technical aspects (e.g., user profiles, data flows, data holders), security implications, and in particular its cultural elements around privacy in a given context. Privacy Impact Assessment (PIA) is a pragmatic manner to make such an analysis. This method was encouraged or made mandatory by various legal frameworks for privacy and data protection in different regions like New Zealand, Canada, Australia, Hong Kong, European Union, (Ericsson et al., 2018). While there is no internationally accepted definition for PIA, the following two definitions are taken into consideration: [PIA is] a process whereby the potential impacts and implications of proposals that involve potential privacy-invasiveness are surfaced and examined (Ericsson et al., 2018). Alternatively, a more detailed construction: A privacy impact assessment as a methodology for assessing the impacts on the privacy of a project, policy, program, service, product, or other initiative and, in consultation with stakeholders, for taking remedial actions as necessary to avoid or minimize negative impacts. A PIA is more than a tool: it is a process that should begin at the earliest possible stages when there are still opportunities to influence the outcome of a project. It is a process that should continue even after the project has been deployed (Abdmeziem and Tandjaoui, 2014).

PIAs can be tailored to a specific technology and application. For instance, Groce and Katz (2010) developed an RFID PIA framework which is used by industry players. Such an approach creates a PIA template that is pertinent to a specific industry sector. Groce and Katz (2010) suggested a PIA template which establishes a four-stage process

(1) A full description of the application and scenario;

(2) Identification of privacy threats;

(3) A proposal of technical and organizational mitigating measures; and

(4) Document the resolution (results of the analysis) regarding the application.

In the same way, m-Health developers could benefit from PIA templates.

1.3.8 Data Anonymization and Obfuscation

High-quality health care requires data sharing (Kouicem et al., 2018). Access control is one of the straightforward strategies to enforce the confidentiality of patients information in health systems. However, we believe that besides the typical binary decision of revealing or not a data value, access control can be further improved with data obfuscation, i.e., for bringing down the accuracy of an individual data item in a controlled, systematic as well as a statistically rigorous manner for guaranteeing the privacy of the patient at the same time preserving its worth (Ouaddah et al., 2017). For instance, instead of revealing the patients age, one can reveal a range of values. Alternatively, one can replace the medical condition or disease with a more general term (e.g., Human Immuno deficiency Virus (HIV) infection replaced by Infectious Disease).

Besides, individuals health information is also important to create rich statistical databases for researchers and to support public health programs. In such cases, data anonymization should be employed, i.e., to protect privacy by making several data transformations so that individuals described by the data remain anonymous. Abdmeziem and Tandjaoui (2014) suggested that the anonymization process can have varying degrees of robustness depending on how likely it : 1) singles out an individual in the data set; 2) links records concerning the same individual; or, 3) infers the value of one attribute based on other values. In essence, all these circumstances should be avoided, resulting in an anonymized data set. Therefore, anonymized data are not considered personal data, so that data privacy laws would no longer be applicable.

1.4 Problem Statement

This work focused on developing the security and privacy mechanisms for the medical IoT. Authentication is the mechanism of identity verification of the entity. Authorization is the mechanism of providing permission to perform some action by the entities. The authorization is performed after the authentication process because after verifying the entity, the algorithms decide whether to grant or deny the access. Authentication and authorization play a major role in security and privacy. There is a difference between the IoT domain and the IT sector. The authentication and authorization cannot be applied directly to the IoT (ContiMauro et al., 2018; Trnka et al., 2017; Kouicem et al., 2018).

Several design challenges are mentioned in the literature. Some of these challenges include the question to what extent the solution should be centralized (i.e. where the decision for allowing or denying access is made) (Ouaddah et al., 2017), what model or which mechanisms, technologies, and protocols to use. Which architecture or solution is most secure or privacy preserving? How to deal with limited computational resources of IoT devices and find smart trade-offs between privacy, security, and technical feasibility? Existing solutions have their own advantages and disadvantages, but it is unclear which matches the needs of the health care sector the most. Ouaddah et al., 2017 mention the dilemma between adapting existing solutions or creating new ones with IoT specific requirements in mind as one of the main open issues for authentication and authorization within the IoT.

1.5 Scope of the Research

All the existing authentication and authorization schemes developed are quite successful to a certain extent, but certain limitations persist while using those methods. Based on their performance analysis, it can be deduced that these methods sometimes cause energy exhaustion of sensor devices and also impose computational overhead on the network. To overcome the above mentioned consequences of using complex authentication and authorization protocols, it is recommended to choose proper authentication and authorization protocols to improve the performance of sensor devices in the system.

1.6 Objectives

The major objectives of the thesis are given below:

1. To deliver mutual authentication solution and thereby minimize the number of mes-

sages to be exchanged. Make it lightweight by adopting simple operations in order to minimize the consumption of resources in the network.

2. To design an authentication protocol for resource-constrained sensor networks, which are the underlying technology of Internet of Things applications.

3. To evaluate the resistance of the protocols against the known active and passive attacks in the perception layer of IoT.

4. To compute various performance metrices like computation time, communication overhead of the devised protocol and compare against other existing protocols.

1.7 Thesis Contribution and Organization

The main contributions of this Thesis are:

(i) Identifying the security requirements for data transmission in IoT;

(ii) Identifying the suitable authentication protocols for the medical IoT and

(iii) Presenting known privacy and security solutions for the medical IoT.

Additionally chapter 1 explains the introduction of IoT, Medical IoT, and communication patterns in IoT, the motivation towards the authentication and authorization problems in IoT, and the objectives of the research are discussed.

Chapter 2 reviews the related work regarding the authentication and authorization mechanism to meet the privacy and security requriements in Medical-IoT.

Chapter 3 deals with the secure data transmission mechanism for M-IoT. It contains modules of a generation of the symmetric key, authentication and disjoint multipath data transmission. The authentication module validates the gateways with the cloud data servers. The symmetric key generation generates the public key for encryption and decryption. The disjoint multipath data transmission divides the encrypted data into fragments and sends it to the server.

Chapter 4 explains the architecture to manage the voluminous data related to the medical field produced by the sensor nodes. The architecture provides secure communication to share data between doctors and patients during ordinary as well as emergency situations.

Chapter 5 deals with the mechanisms of authentication of various kinds among the patients as well as doctors located in distant geographical areas. The mechanism, in the proposal offers the integrity of data, privacy as well as mutual authentication. In addition, it utilizes the methods of symmetric encryption for preserving the security in M-IoT.
Finally, Chapter 6 concludes the research work by comparing the proposed models.

CHAPTER 2

LITERATURE SURVEY

IoT by definition is what connects any things like devices to people or things such as embedded sensors containing software at any place via the internet at any time. Health care is one of the most trending areas for IoT. The IoT is used in many applications like remote monitoring, disabled and elderly care, treating patients at home through telemedicine, etc. Therefore many sensor nodes and smart devices act as the core devices in the IoT. Health care IoT improves the patients life and has the objective to reduce the implementation cost. Figure 2.1 shows the framework of health care IoT. IoT provides cost-effective communication among sensor nodes, patients, doctors, health care centers and hospitals.

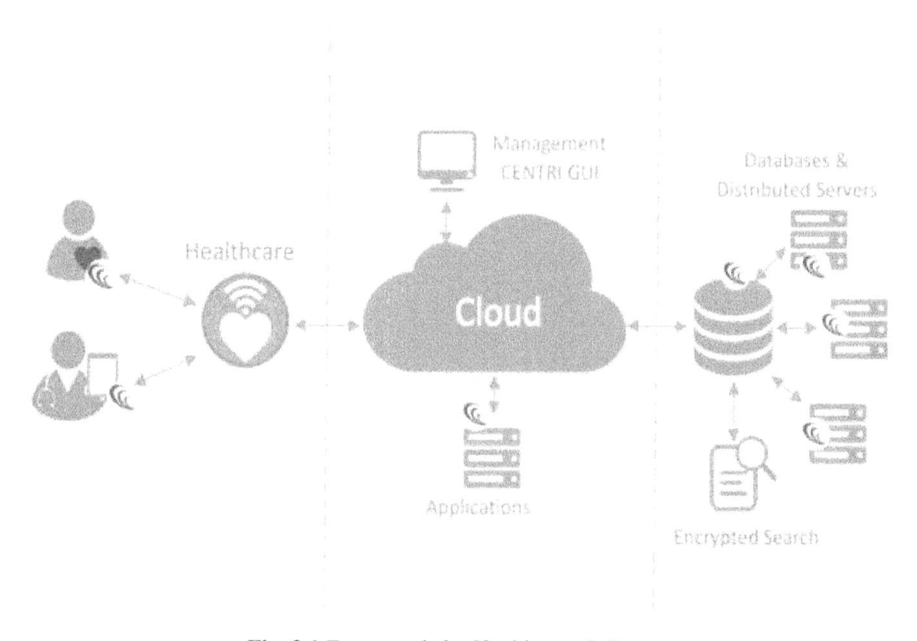

Fig. 2.1 Framework for Health care IoT

The devices like gateways, middle layer services, and databases play a crucial role in managing health care records and also they are helpful in providing on-demand services to the stakeholders.
For the past decade, health care IoT is attracting many researchers to concentrate on different issues in health care and IoT. Based on this, there are several architectures, protocols and frameworks available in the health care IoT field. Many research contributions in health care IoT focused on developing the architectures, platforms, security, and interoperability among other services. However, there are still challenges in the health care IoT field that need to be addressed. This chapter focuses on the recent advancements in the health care IoT and identifies challenges to incorporating health care into IoT.

2.1 IoT Network in Health care

The IoT network was considered a crucial part of health care IoT. The IoT network facilitated sending and receiving of the data related to medical work from the sensor nodes towards the base station and also enabled communication between all the IoT devices. Figure 2.2 shows the topology of the IoT networks which was discussed in detail in (Zhu et al., 2010; Gronbaek 2008).

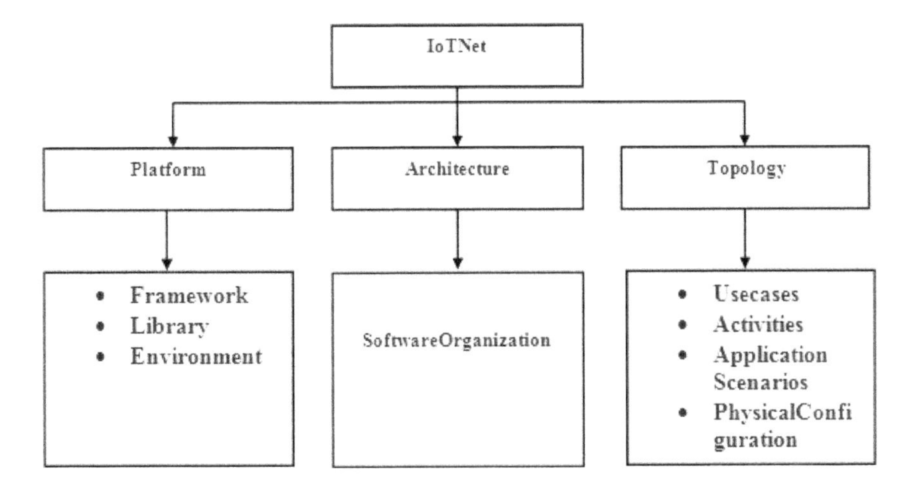

Fig. 2.2 IoT Network Topology

2.1.1 IoT Net

The topologies in the IoT Net refer to the integration of different services into the health care IoT environment. Figure 2.3 explains the heterogeneous cloud environment where it collects medical data from different sensors like temperature, blood pressure, Electrocardiograms. The cloud environment provides the computing infrastructure for devices like smartphones, laptops, and medical centers (Viswanathan et al., 2010).

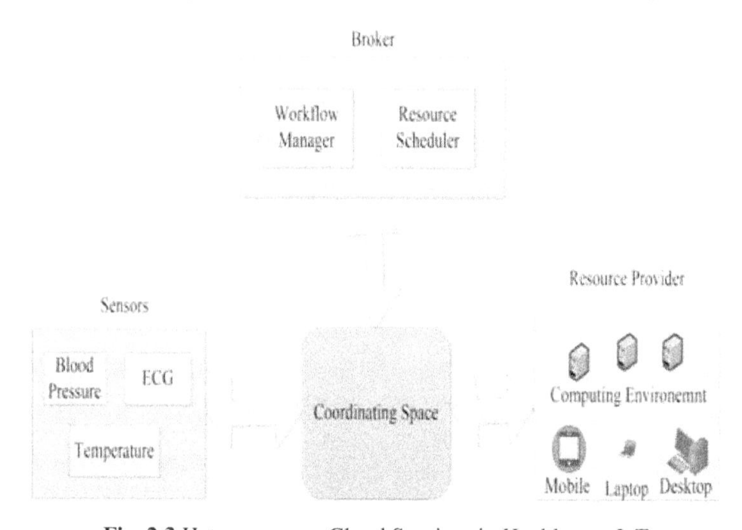

Fig. 2.3 Heterogeneous Cloud Services in Health care IoT

Figure 2.4 shows the remote health care monitoring system using sensor nodes attached to the patients body. The sensor nodes record, analyze and store data from different sensor nodes which is later aggregated for further use. The doctors or health centers could access this aggregated data from anywhere and anytime to treat the patients accordingly. With respect to this, the network topology includes the network structure to support video streaming. For instance, the WiMAX, GSM, IP are the network structures used to access the ultrasound videos (Zhao et al., 2011; Yang et al., 2012; Imadal et al., 2012).

2.2 IoT Network Architecture

The architectures of IoT Net are majorly focused on the physical elements and their working procedures. Figure 2.5 shows the health care IoT along with the ambient assistant model (Istepanian, 2011). This architecture discusses the interoperability of the WLAN, WPAN and Multimedia streaming, Health care centers, and IoT gateways. In

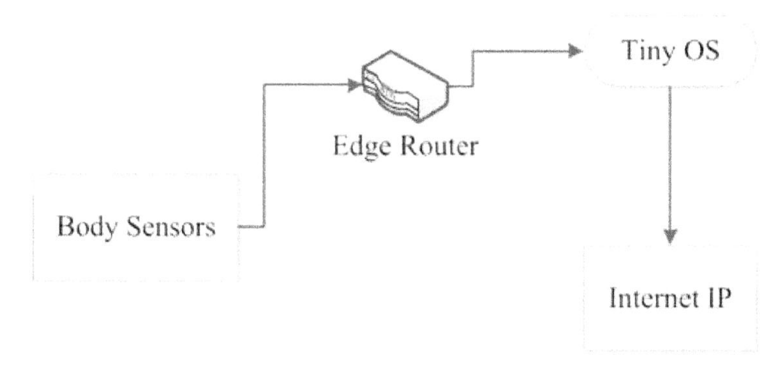

Fig. 2.4 Remote Health care Monitoring System

the recent studies, authors have justified the IPV6 based WPAN as the base for the IoT network (Zhang, 2011; Shahamabadi et al., 2013; Jara et al., 2010; Istepanian et al., 2011; Bui et al., 2010).

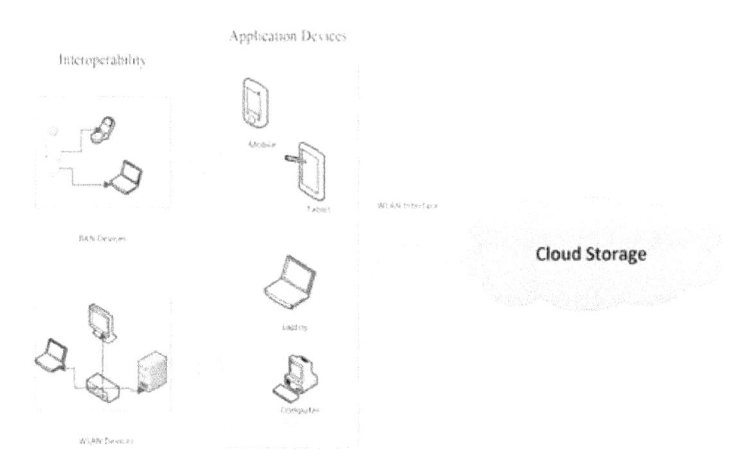

Fig. 2.5 IoT Network Architecture for Health care and Ambient Assistance

Figure 2.6 shows the layered architecture of the WLAN. In the IoT Network, the IoT devices and sensor nodes used the IPV6 for data transmission. Then the reply from the sensor nodes is done through the UDP packets. The WLAN has some limitations in the health care IoT. It cannot support mobility in the network.

To address the mobility in the health care IoT, four approaches are considered (Bui et al., 2010) which include the directed acyclic graph information object (DIO) that is attached to the patients to send the messages. You et al. (2011), proposed a gateway protocol to address mobility in health care IoT. This protocol addressed the periodic traffic, query-driven traffic, and abnormal traffic which could be managed in the heterogeneous network. Swiatek and Rucinsk (2013) proposed an e-health mechanism with three complex modules composition, signaling, and transmission.

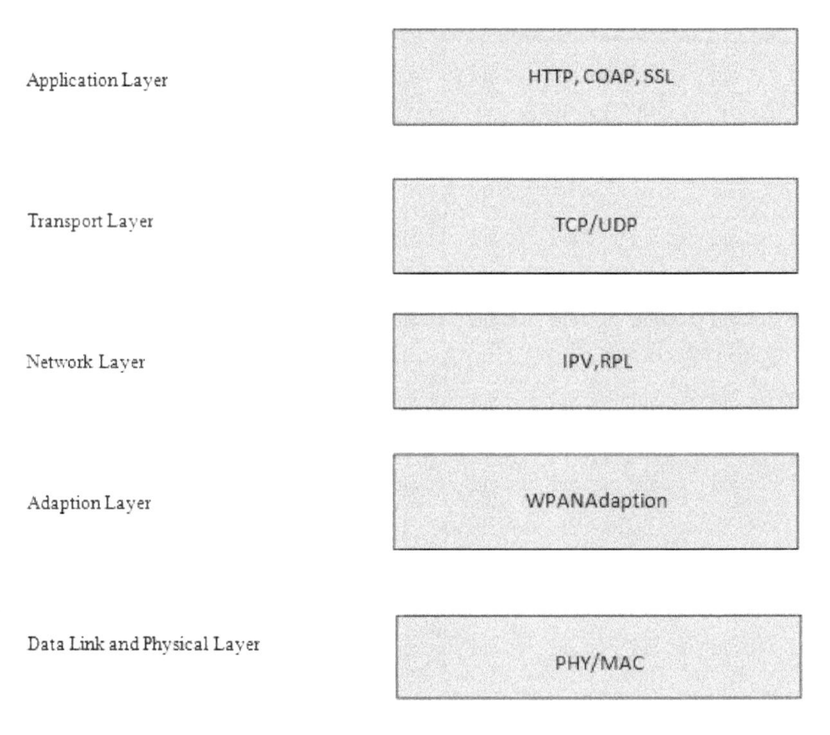

Fig. 2.6 Layered Architecture of WLAN in Health care IoT

2.3 Applications and Services of Health care IoT

Health care based IoT environment can have many different applications in different fields like elderly and pediatric patients, health and fitness management, and monitoring of chronic diseases. This research work classifies Health care IoT applications into two sets. One is related to single condition applications like treating specific diseases and the other deals with the number of diseases. Figure 2.7 shows the health care IoT applications and services that are available in todays world.

2.3.1 Health care IoT Applications

The health care IoT applications are directly used by the patients and doctors and it is a user-centric mechanism in ECG Monitoring, glucose level sensing, blood pressure monitoring, temperature sensing, medication monitoring, and smartphone health care. In chronic conditions on-time alert is very critical and important. The M-IoT devices collect all signs of diseases and send data to doctors for tracking patients in real time. Ingestible sensors are used by diabetic patients as it is used in identifying symptoms and giving patients an early warning messages when they are in critical position.
ECG Monitoring: The electrocardiogram monitoring is also an application of health care IoT which records the heart rate of patients and forwards the data to the storage purpose. Many researchers developed algorithms for IoT based ECG sensing (Yang et al., 2014; Castillejo et al., 2013; Agu et al., 2013). Liu et al., (2012) developed the IoT based ECG sensing model by using the portable sensor with transmitter and wireless receiver. The proposed approach uses the search automation method to identify the abnormalities in the patients real-time data.

Glucose Level Sensing: The monitoring of glucose levels in diabetes patients helps them to modify their diet plans, meditation, and activities. Istepanian et al., (2011) configured the M- IoT to monitor glucose levels on a real-time basis. This method used the IPv6 protocol to transmit the sensing data to the health care providers.
Blood Pressure Sensing: Dohr et al., (2010) proposed a combined KIT BP meter with NFC enabled KIT smartphone to monitor the blood pressure using the IoT. Puustjarvi and Puustjarvi (2011) developed the communication structure to transmit the BP sensing data to the users as well as the health care centers.
Temperature Monitoring: Monitoring body temperature is a crucial part of health care services. The body temperature is an important sign for homeostasis maintenance. Ruiz et al., (2009) proposed the concept of M- IoT using the body temperature sensor. The results showed the variations in the body temperature which successfully integrated with the M- IoT. Jian et al., (2012) proposed the temperature-based M- IoT model using the home gateway .
Medication Monitoring: Pang et al., (2014) developed the IoT based medication monitoring system to provide an intelligent packaging method. This method used i- MedBox which controlled the packing mechanism of medicines to avoid noncompliance problems. Laranjo et al., (2012) proposed the RFID based architecture for e-health over IoT.
Smartphone Health care: In recent years, smartphone usage in the IoT environment has increased rapidly. Many software and hardware devices are used to design the health care environment using a smartphone. Mosa et al., (2012), discussed the different health care applications using smartphones. This survey included research on health care apps,

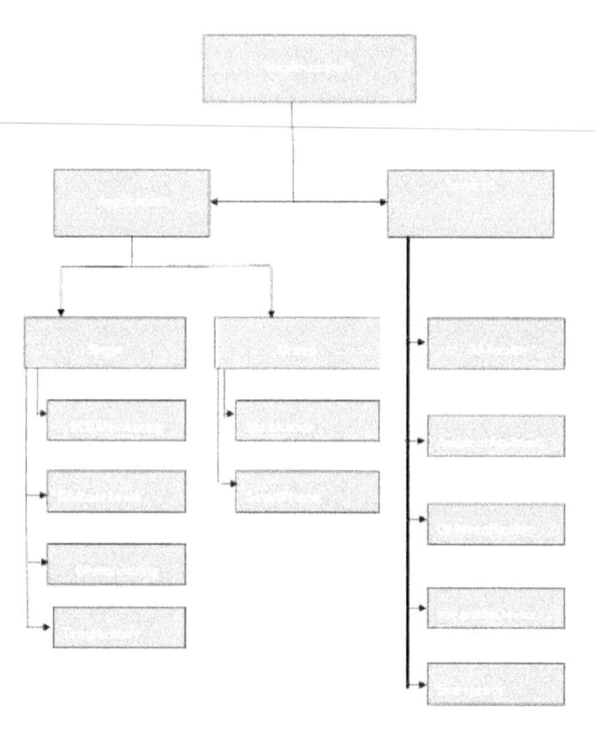

Fig. 2.7 Health care IoT Applications and Services

training apps, search apps, and other health-related apps. Figure 2.8 shows the classification of smartphone health care apps.

2.3.2 Health care IoT Services

The IoT is enabled with a different type of health care services where each service provides a different type of health care. The services like m-health, ambient assistant living, childrens health services, wearable device access, and emergency health care are discussed below.

Mobile-Health IoT: As shown in Istepanian et al., (2012) the m-health contains the sensor nodes, mobile computing, communication technologies for the health care environment. The m-health environment provides a new health care environment which uses the WPAN with 4G network for internet based m-health. The major challenge faced by the m-health environment is context aware issues. Ambient Assistant Living: The IoT based health care services support the elderly people services. The IoT platform

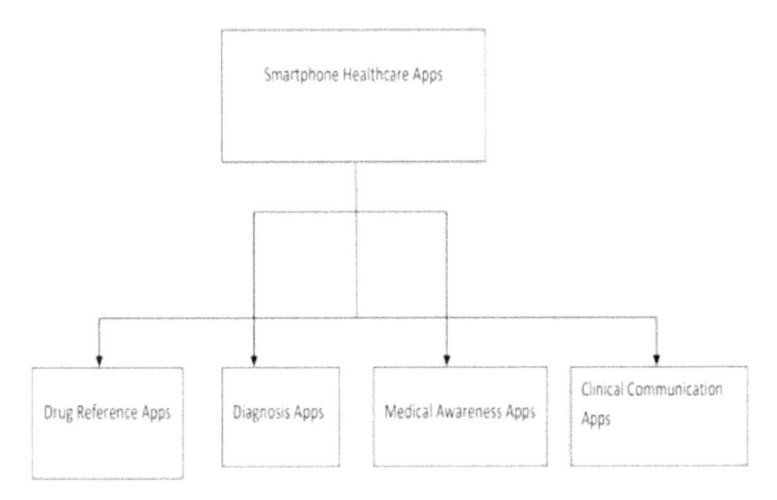

Fig. 2.8 Classifications of Smartphone Health care Apps

which is combined with artificial intelligence to assist the elderly and disabled people is called ambient assistant living (AAL). The main aim of AAL is to provide comfort living to the elderly and disabled people. Shahamabadi et al., (2013) proposed architecture for security control, automation, and communication. This architecture provides health care services to the disabled and elderly people.

Children Health Service:The investigation of childrens health like mental behavior is crucial to gather information globally. Many researchers have concentrated on developing the IoT service for gathering childrens health information. M. VazquezBriseno et al., (2014) developed an IoT based m-health to monitor childrens activities with the help of their parents and teachers.

Access to Wearable Devices:Many sensors are developed to assist medical applications. The same sensors have been used to access the IoT services on one hand, while on the other end, wearable devices came into the picture with better features for IoT architecture. Bazzani et al., (2012) developed the IoT based activity monitoring model using wearable devices. They used Bluetooth technology to connect with IoT technology.

Emergency Health care: Emergency situations like accidents, earthquakes, weather conditions and fire accidents involve many health care issues. In these types of situation, health care services can offer different solutions like alerts, post-accident action, and data storage (Xiao et al., 2013).

2.4 Security and Privacy in Health care IoT

Many organizations donot spend resources to provide security and privacy in health care (Huang et al., 2018). But security and privacy play a crucial role in health care IoT. The health care IoT produces large volumes of sensor data which are more sensitive. Privacy is more crucial in all stages of medical IoT like data collection, transmission, storage, and retrieval. To provide security and privacy to the M- IoT, the following should be considered

- Data Usability
- Data Integrity
- Data Auditing
- Data Privacy

Data Usability: It is defined as the process of ensuring the data being accessed by authorized users. The data in the M- IoT have great advantages along with major issues like raw data and unfiltered data. With respect to this, data loss or corruption leads to the restriction of data usability.

Data Integrity: It is defined as the process of satisfying the data values with standards and not giving scope to data tampering. The data integrity is categorized into user-defined integrity, referential integrity, domain integrity, and entity integrity.

Data Auditing: The auditing of medical data is crucial to find the accessibility of the resources and it is also helpful in finding abnormal activities. The medical data is stored in third-party servers. So the M- IoT requires suitable auditing mechanisms.

Patients data privacy: The patients data is classified into two types: general and sensitive data. The sensitive records contain the patients information like mental status, disease description, genetic information, drug addiction, identity information, and sexual information. It is important to preserve privacy of the patients data.

Many M- IoT devices are limited with memory, battery power, and computing capacity, so they require additional support for power supply, memory, and high-scale computing for real-time data processing and storage. In recent trends, the cloud environment is extensively used in processing and storing of medical data.

2.4.1 Data Encryption

Data encryption is one of the methods where it provides security to the data in the communication process with a set of rules (Zhao, 2016). Figure 2.9 represents the data encryption mechanism where the plain text is converted into ciphertext using an encryption algorithm. The public key or private key is used to decrypt the text. In general, the encryption process is performed in three stages of communication: end-to-end encryption process, link encryption process and node encryption process.

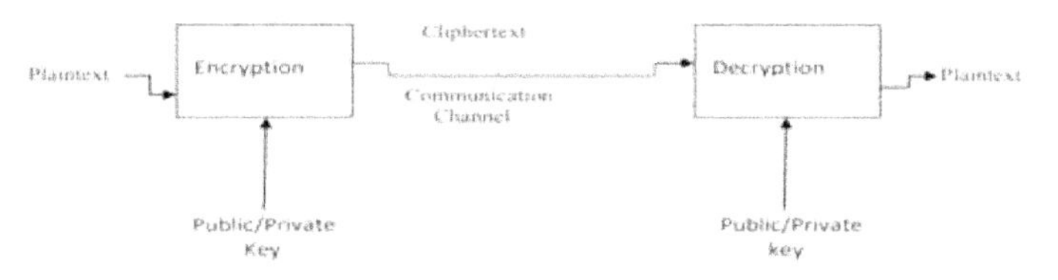

Fig. 2.9 Data Encryption and Decryption Process

The end-to-end encryption is the process of transmitting the encrypted message and it cannot be decrypted until it reaches the destination. In the link encryption, at the end of each link, the intermediate nodes decrypt the message into plain text and again plain text is converted into cipher text using the secret key. The node encryption process will not allow the plain text to transmit into the network. The node encryption process is a highly secure mechanism.

To provide security to the M- IoT, secret key management plays a crucial role. Moreover, the transmission protocols or encryption algorithms highly affect the transmission rate of the network and also sometimes they lead to failure in data transmission. Table 2.1 shows some of the encryption algorithms which are used in the M- IoT.

The medical IoT devices have limited resources and lead to many challenges in the security and privacy of e-Health applications. Abdmeziem and Tandjaoui (2014) developed the lightweight key management algorithm which would consume fewer resources in the key exchange. In this proposed work, the heterogeneous network is considered where the nodes have different resource capabilities. Efficient encryption algorithms and symmetric key generation algorithms require nodes with high computational capacity. So the proposed method considered the offloading capacity to upload the symmetric generation mechanism to the third-party service providers.

Gong et al., (2015) developed the lightweight homomorphism algorithms which considered the characteristics of privacy protection in the IoT environment. The authors designed a simulation environment using hardware and software to prove the proposed

Table 2.1 Data Encryption Algorithms for M-IoT

Encryption Algorithms	**Advantages**	**Applications**
Light weight key management algorithm (Abdmeziem and Tandjaoui,2014)	Over comes the issues of limited computing capacity using efficient authentication mechanisms	Used in source-constrained nodes
Homomorphism Algorithm(Gong etal., 2015)	Efficient encryption process which considers the properties of IoT	For efficient data transmission in IoT
Asymmetric Encryption Algorithm (Huetal.,2017)	Minimizes the consumption of medical resources	For securing the data of elderly and disabled people
Key Agreement Algorithm	Improves the Authenticity	Emergency health care

method. Hu et al., (2017) developed the model based on IoT and cloud environment which will focus on digital signatures, certifications, and time stamps and asymmetric encryption mechanisms. They provide security to the health care services to the disabled and elderly people.
Li et al., (2016) proposed the authentication mechanism for wireless body area networks which considered the cloud as a platform to implement key agreement protocol using chaotic maps. Figure 2.10 shows the architecture of the cloud-assisted WBAN.

The Diffie-Hellman algorithm for the exchange of key is used by the participants to register into the network. The data collected from the WBAN sensors will be encrypted and forwarded to the gateway and again from the gateway to the cloud. The health care professionals and patients can access the data from a cloud environment to analyze and upload the data again.

2.4.2 Access Control Mechanisms

Access Control Mechanisms defined as the process of identifying the user identity and granting permission to authorized users (Bacis et al., 2016). There are different types of encryption mechanisms that are used in the access control such as Attribute-Based Encryption (ABE), Asymmetric Key Encryption (AKE), and Symmetric key Encryption (SKE) (Goyal et al., 2006). In general, cryptography is performed using the keys. The size of the key and mechanism used will directly reflect the performance of the encryption and decryption. Hence, the cryptographic life cycle depend on the key man-

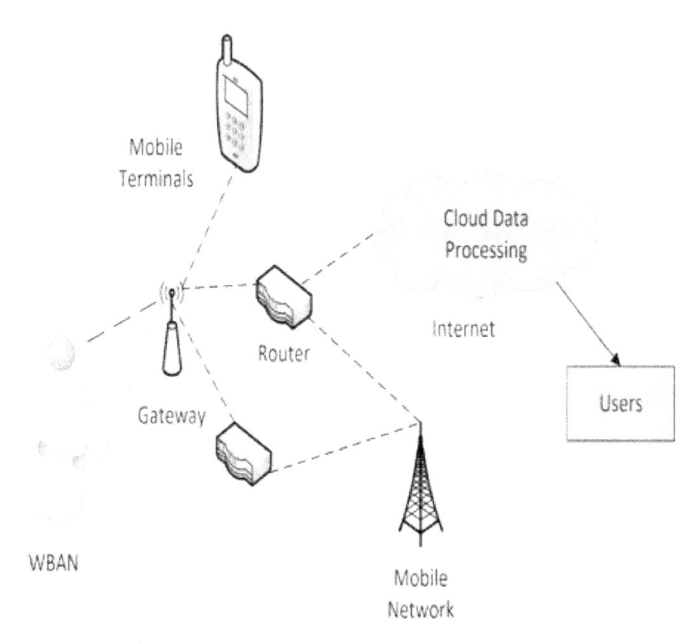

Fig. 2.10 Architecture for cloud-assisted WBAN

agement schemes. For instance, ABE is one of the mechanisms which has efficient key management schemes. Table 2.2 shows the existing access control mechanisms.

In health care data exchange, patient records can be shared through the internet or intranet by providing authorization for data exchange. But, the existing authorization mechanism has different challenges in reaching the needs of the health care data exchange for not having the security and policy mechanisms. Bethencourt et al., (2007) developed the authorization mechanisms for cloud based health care data exchange which overcame the drawbacks of the cryptographic and non-cryptographic approaches. Figure 2.11 shows the cryptographic approach in health care organizations. The proposed framework consists of the Health care data exchange cloud, health care authorities and patients. Bethencourt et al., (2007) developed a signature based algorithm along with a hashing scheme to authorize and authenticate the patients to grant permission to access the cloud for data exchange. Based on their assumption, the proposed proxy based hashing mechanism achieved privacy and security.

Lounis et al., (2013) developed the architecture based on ABE algorithms which is given in Figure 2.12. It is observed that the access permission is revoked when the emergency work is completed. Here, the revoking of access rights is very difficult in ABE

Table 2.2 Access Control Mechanisms in Cryptography

Algorithms	Advantages	Applications
Attribute-Based Encryption (Lounis et al.,2013)	Used to solve there vocation issue	To perform access control
Cipher text Policy based ABE (Hadjidj etal., 2016)	To manage the dynamic and complex policies	Used in medical networks
ABE in patient-centric frame work(Li etal., 2012)	To encrypt patient health records	To perform access control to the patient health records

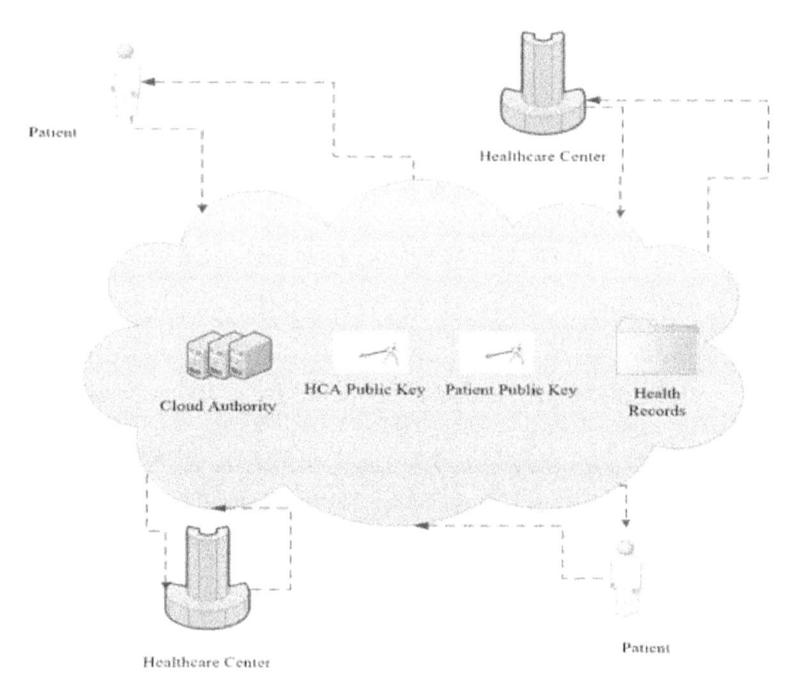

Fig. 2.11 Cryptographic Approach in Health care Organization

algorithms and it causes a high computation load. Bethencourt et al., (2007) used integer comparisons to resolve the revocation issue. With respect to this, they proposed the numerical attribute to find the expiry time emergency key. The experimental analysis proved that the proposed method achieved less revocation cost and an efficient access control mechanism.

Lounis et al., (2016) developed the cloud based architecture for WBANs and proposed the access policies for dynamic privacy which used the CP-ABE algorithm. The experimental results proved that the proposed access policies are efficient and scalable. Li et al., (2012) proposed the framework for health care. They proposed the access policies for accessing the patient records from the cloud. The authors used ABE algorithms to encrypt the patients health records and preserve the privacy of patients.

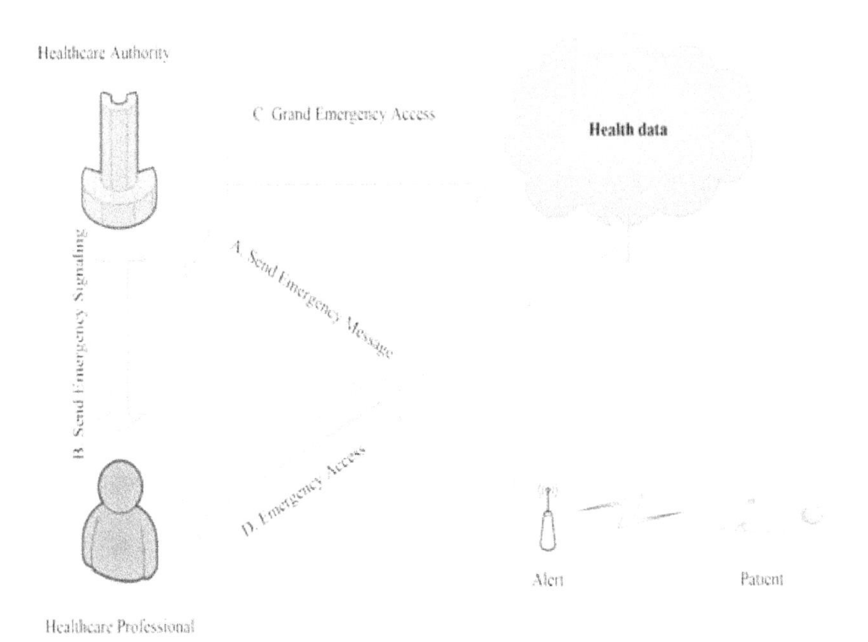

Fig. 2.12 Architecture for Emergency Access Control

The access and privacy controls are personalized to the virtualized resources that are distributed over the network. Unauthorized access to virtualized resources is a serious risk, which compromises linked user privacy. At disparate time instances, the access control process depends upon the virtualized resource's states and privacy preserving relies upon the service response's longevity. For enhancing service-related performance, access delegation along with denial was determined by the conversion of the resource's states as assisted by the Q-learning process. By metrics like true positives, access time, as well as alteration, access denial, and also success ratio, memory utilization, along with time complexity, the performance for accessing control along with privacy, was verified. For saving the data, the blockchain centred approach occupies more space.

Ostad-Sharif et al recommended a safe and lightweight authentication together with a key agreement protocol aimed at IoT centred wireless sensor networks (WSN) that was free of the former protocol's security problems. The system setup, registration, login as well as verification, along with password change phases are the four phases of the protocol. The famous and extensively approved Automated Validation of Internet Security Protocols and also Applications tool introduced the protocol's formal security verification. The protocol's superiority was denoted by the comparative security along with performance assessments with other associated works . The efficiency level was tested only with fewer sensor nodes or machines, so its efficiency was not dependable.

2.4.3 Third-Party Auditing

In the health care IoT, cloud servers play a crucial role in storing health records. The cloud servers are managed by third parties who are not fully trusted. The cloud servers would be compromised and the medical data can meddle without the users permission. The user specifies the rules to access the health care data and the cloud service provider does not have the right to access the data. To protect the rights of the users, third-party auditing is required to monitor the activity of the CSPs (Venkatesh and Parthasarathi, 2013). The major challenges of the third party are batch auditing, dynamic auditing and performance auditing.

In recent years, many aproaches were proposed for third-party auditing. The algorithms like support vector machine and logic regression are proposed for finding suspicious actions on the servers. In the present trend, unsupervised learning algorithms are used for auditing purposes (Boxwala et al., 2011).

Chen et al., (2012) developed the approach about relational learning of the boss as well as the colleagues for developing networks to interact at departments level. The authors proposed two mechanisms to divide the department interactions. Govaert et al., (2015) surveyed audits and operational costs relationship. Based on the authors study, surgical auditing is defined as the quality metric and they further continued their investigation to reduce the cost.

2.4.4 Data Search Algorithms

To provide privacy, the medical data should be encrypted before it is stored in the cloud environment. This approach will obstruct the traditional keyword search methods. Therefore, developing the encryption based keyword search is required in the cloud (Cao et al., 2011). Some of the algorithms are Public Key Encryption with Searchable approach (PEKS) and Symmetric encryption with Searchable mechanism (SSK) and it is to be noted that the algorithms that has complex procedure lead to difficulty in searching.

Table 2.3 Data Searching Algorithms in Cloud Environment

Algorithms	Advantages	Applications
attribute-based multi-keyword search(Miao etal.,2016)	Having better edges estimation with edges information	Applied over encrypted images
Symmetric key based Approach (Bezawada etal.,2015)	Having efficient privacy mechanism to protect from semi honest attacks	It uses string matching for preserving the privacy
Authorized private keyword Searches(Li etal.,2011)	It supports multi-keyword Search	Applied over patients health records
Laplace guided kernel regression method (Song etal., 2013)	It grants permissions to users to access the localized servers based on their attributes	Applied over patients health records

In the present trend, to overcome the resource burden and improve the resource capacity, patients health records are migrating gradually towards the storage of the cloud. Miao et al., (2016) developed the attribute pivoted multi-keyword searching algorithm across the medical records with encryption in the cloud environment. This method supports multi-keyword search in CP-ABE and also provides fine-grained access control. Figure 2.13 shows the attribute based multi-keyword search algorithm. The experimental results proved the efficiency of the search mechanism.

Bezawada et al., (2015) designed the method of the symmetric key pivoted encryption to secure privacy in the cloud environment. The authors designed a pattern search algorithm which is an efficient indexing structure. This indexing mechanism uses the balanced binary tree structure to find the keyword similarities. Figure 2.14 shows the indexing mechanism and also develops the algorithm to find the rank to retrieve the documents of relevance based on the clients query.

Li et al., (2011) addressed the problem of search using keywords across health records with encryption. The proposed model grants permission to the users with the help of a third party based on the user attributes. This model provides the query and document privacy along with multi-keyword search. Song et al., (2013) developed the kernel regression algorithm to restore the images with a less computational cost. The Laplace kernel method is used for smoothing kernel for kernel regression.

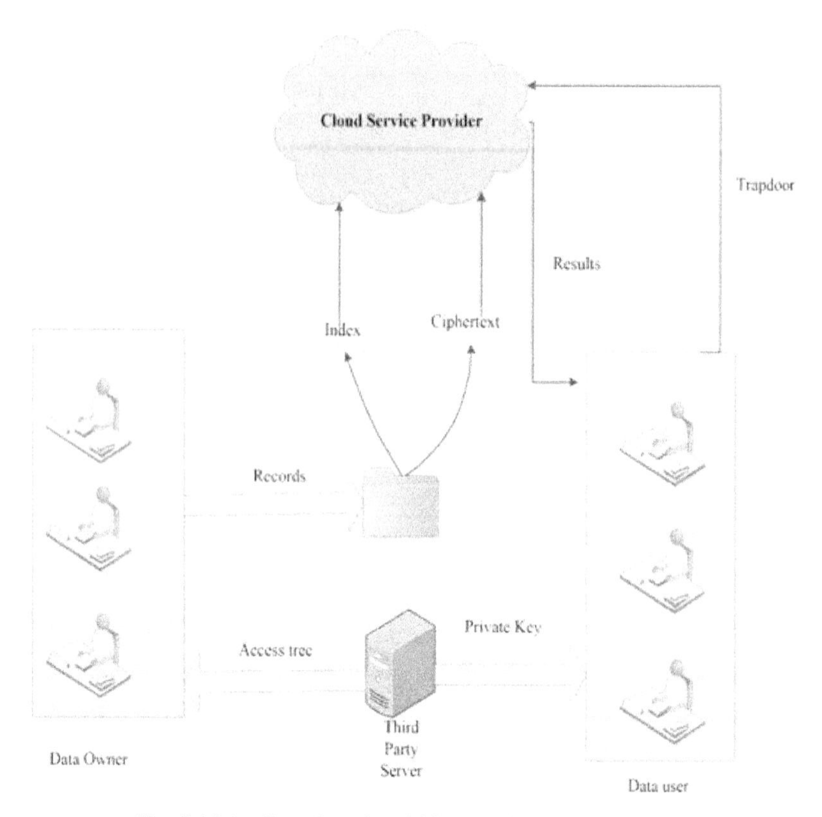

Fig. 2.13 Attribute based multi-keyword Search Algorithm

2.4.5 Data Anonymization

Medical data is categorized into three modules such as privacy attributes, quasi identifiers and explicit identifiers. Privacy attributes refer to the important information of the patients like income and disease description. The quasi identifiers are represented with age, date of birth, address. The explicit identifiers refer to the identity of the patient like the name, patient ID as well as phone number.To protect patient privacy, each attribute needs to be properly addressed in the distribution data. In the present trend, to solve the issues of anonymity, many algorithms are proposed such as l-diversity, k-anonymity, and confidence bounding. In particular, k-anonymity is widely used in the privacy-preserving approaches. But, K-anonymity is not sufficient to deal with sensitive data. Attacks like knowledge attacks and consistency attacks access sensitive data

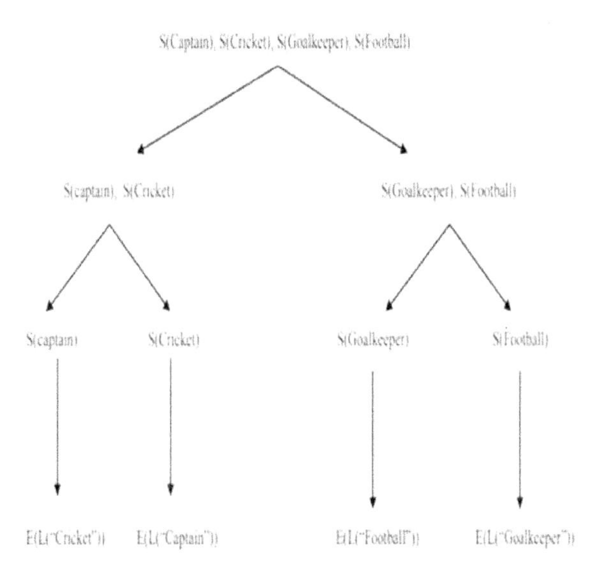

Fig. 2.14 Indexing Mechanism

which causes severe damage to data privacy.

Miao et al., (2016) identified three issues such as the utility of data, high dimensionality and algorithm which restrict the usage of conventional anonymization algorithms over the sensitive data. The authors proposed the LKC model for privacy using two different algorithms such as distribution and centralized anonymization algorithms. Adult and blood databases are the two real-time data sets that are used for experimentation. The outcomes establish that the algorithm in the proposal has the capability in handling the privacy of sensitive data.

Many algorithms have been employed for k-anonymization to perform data anonymization. With respect to longitudinal information, the major issue is to identify the distance metrics. Figure 2.15 shows the architecture of the anonymization process in longitudinal information.

Fung et al., (2010) proposed the MDAV algorithm for k-anonymity to perform the clustering process. The proposed method selected the highest trajectory from the data set to form the cluster for k-records. Liu and Li (2018) developed the clustering method for k-anonymity for preserving the privacy of medical devices. The k-anonymity clustering approach groups the same records into a similar set. Quasi identifiers are used to

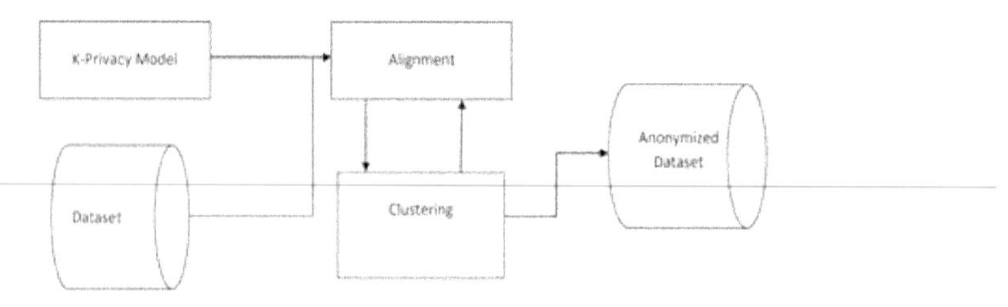

Fig. 2.15 Architecture of Anonymization Process in Longitudinal Information

suppress and generalize the operations.

2.5 Security Challenges in Health care IoT

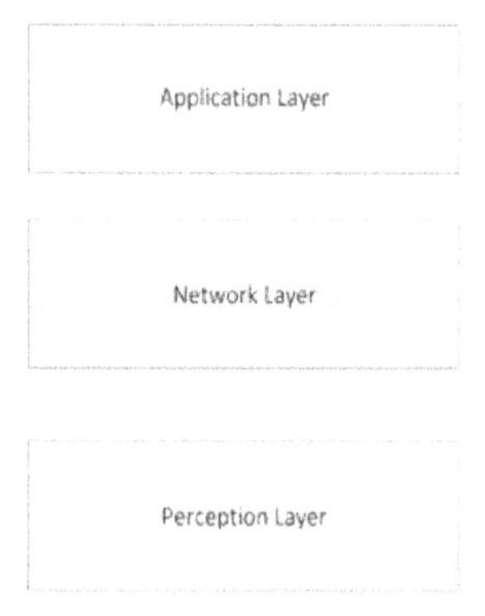

Fig. 2.16 Security Reference Architecture for Health care IoT

The security reference architecture for IoT consists of three layers which are shown in Figure 2.16 (Weyrich and Ebert, 2016; Bauer et al., 2013)

Perception layer: This layer is associated with a physical layer that fetches the information from different sensors like temperature, speed, humidity, and location.

Network layer: This layer fetches the information from the perception layer and forwards it to the application layer through different communication technologies like Bluetooth, ZigBee, Wi-Fi, 3G, 4G, and 5G networks.

Application layer: The layer has the responsibility to deliver the service that is application specific towards clients. Some of the security services in health care IoT and some other security concerns are described below:

- Authentication
- Authorization
- Confidentiality
- Integrity
- Non-Repudiation
- Availability
- Privacy

a) Authentication: Process of validating the identity of the user. In the IoT perspective, each object/ thing needs to be identified or validated from all the things/objects in the network.

b) Authorization: Process of granting permission to the user to do some action.

c) Confidentiality: Process of guaranteeing that the data should be accessed only by authorized users.

d) Integrity: Process of satisfying the data values with standards and not giving scope to data tampering. The data integrity is categorized into user defined integrity, referential integrity, domain integrity, and entity integrity.

e) Non-Repudiation: Process of ensuring the action has occurred which cannot be later denied by the user.

f) Availability: Process of guaranteeing the service available to respective users at anytime and anywhere.

g) Privacy: Process of guaranteeing the non-accessibility to sensitive data by anyone other than the owner.

2.5.1 Security Challenges in Perception Layer

The perception layer consists of sensor nodes which have limited battery power, computation capacity and memory. Based on these limitations, many attacks have been raised and those are given as follows:

- Denial of Service attack
- Node Capture
- Distributed Denial of Service Attack
- Sybil Attack
- Denial of Sleep attack
- Replay Attack
- Side Channel Attack
- Routing Threats
- Sensor Tracking

a) Denial of Service Attack: This attack would restrict the user to access the resources and terminate the network or system. The DoS attacks occur due to the overwhelming huge quantity of spam requests which overloads and prevents the system to deliver the normal services (Anirudh et al., 2017).

b) Node Capture: These types of attacks are easy for the attackers to compromise the nodes. The attackers capture the nodes and compromise the encryption techniques. They clone the malicious nodes and place them in the network which would compromise the complete security of the network (Zhu et al., 2007).

c) DDoS attack: The advanced version of the DoS attack is a DDoS attack. A major issue is requiring the ability to transfer large traffic from different IoT nodes through the compromised server (Machaka et al., 2016).

d) Sybil Attack: These attacks are concerned with creating fake identities and deploying them using fake nodes. With the help of fake nodes, the attackers generate the fake data and also communicate the spam data to the neighboring nodes (Zhang et al., 2014).

e) Denial of Sleep attack: The IoT sensor nodes have limited battery power, so they would operate the sleep mode to save energy. But the denial of sleep attack increases the power consumption of the nodes which ultimately decreases the nodes lifetime (Uher et al., 2016).

f) Replay Attack:These attacks are commonly used over the authentication mechanism. In these attacks, the data is stored and transmitted without any authority (Na et al., 2017).

g) Side Channel Attack: These attacks are applied over the encryption devices based on the information of hardware to analyze the information like power consumption, execution time, power dissipation, and inference. The attackers use this information to find the secret keys at the time of encryption (Pammu et al., 2016).

h) Routing Threats: These attacks commonly appear in the network layer, but sometimes the attackers employ the routing attacks in the data forwarding phase of the perception layer. These attacks increase the error messages and delay by creating the routing loop (Airehrour et al., 2016).

i) Sensor Tracking: Attackers can make use of real time devices to acwuire patient location, further which violates privacy of patient. GPS Tracking sensors are used in devices to send the location of patient in case of emergency. If device is vulnerable then attacker may spoof GPS data and find patients location.

2.5.2 Security Challenges in Network Layer

The Network layer is responsible for fetching the data from the perception layer and transmitting it to the application layer and it is also responsible for data routing and primary data analysis. This layer uses different communication technologies such as Bluetooth, ZigBee, Wi-Fi, 3G, 4G, and 5G networks. The following are the different challenges faced by the network layer in Health care IoT.

- Man in the Middle Attack
- Denial of Service (DoS)
- Eavesdropping
- Routing Attacks

Man in the Middle Attack: This allows the attackers to listen to the traffic, allows to modify the traffic, and spoof the data at the client and server side. Based on the survey of McAfee, the most attacks are MITM and DDoS ones (Ekerevac et al., 2017).

Denial of Service (DoS): The DoS attacks occur in the network layer which interfere with the transmission signals, using Sybil attacks, affecting the routing process in the network (Airehrour et al., 2016).

Eavesdropping: It is a passive attack where the attacker would listen to the communication over the transmission and also they would extract the information like node configuration, user names, passwords (Mukherjee et al., 2015).

Routing Attacks: The routing attacks are focused on the data routing process. The attackers spoof the messages, sometimes eavesdrop on the packets or redirect the data, in the network layer. Some of the routing attacks are given below:

- Gray Hole (Tseng et al., 2015)
- Black Hole(Xiaopeng et al., 2007)
- Hello Flooding (Ahmed et al., 2016)
- Worm Hole(Sharma et al., 2016)
- Sybil Attack(Nastase et al., 2017)

The above potential attacks require the following security services in the network:

- Point-to-point Authentication
- Hop-to-Hop Encryption
- Intrusion Detection and Secure Routing
- Key Agreement and Management

2.5.3 Security Challenges in the Application layer

Attacks in the application layer, primarily look for unauthorized access to sensitive user information, which violates the privacy of the user. Attackers exploit the advantage of software and device bugs on the application layer to seek the services and applications offered by the layer. It is also responsible for managing many protocols for message passing which are given as follows (Wang et al., 2017; Hedi et al., 2017; Mahmoud et al., 2015).

- Message Queuing Telemetry Transport (MQTT)

- COnstrained Application Protocol (COAP)
- Advanced Message Queuing Protocol (AMQP)
- Extensible Messaging and Presence Protocol (XMPP)

The user can directly access the application layer. The application layer protocol is not suitable for IoT applications. A few challenging issues posed to the application layer in IoT are

- Data Accessibility and Authentication
- Data privacy and identity
- Data Availability

Data Accessibility and Authentication: The IoT applications are accessed by many users. The malicious users could access the application and have a great advantage over the particular system. Therefore, different access permissions and control need to be there for every user (Manyika et al., 2015).

Data Privacy and Identity: The IoT consists of different devices which lead to different protocols for authentication. Therefore, the integration of these protocols is a difficult task to ensure the identity and privacy of the data.

Data Availability: The IoT is connected with many devices that produce a huge volume of data. This will create the overhead on the application to analyze the data. Therefore data availability over the big data is a crucial task that should be provided by the application.

From Table 2.4, it is observed that authentication is the major security principles that should be applied in all layers. In IoT, the authentication is carried between the sensor nodes and gateway, and the gateway is authenticated at the cloud.

2.5.4 Taxonomy of the Authentication protocols in Health care IoT

This subsection deals with the taxonomy of the authentication protocols with different characteristics. In the previous section, it is mentioned that authentication is applied in all layers of the IoT which differentiates the authentication techniques. Figure 2.17 shows the taxonomy of authentication in health care IoT. Table 2.5 shows the advantages and disadvantages of algorithms that are used for authentication.

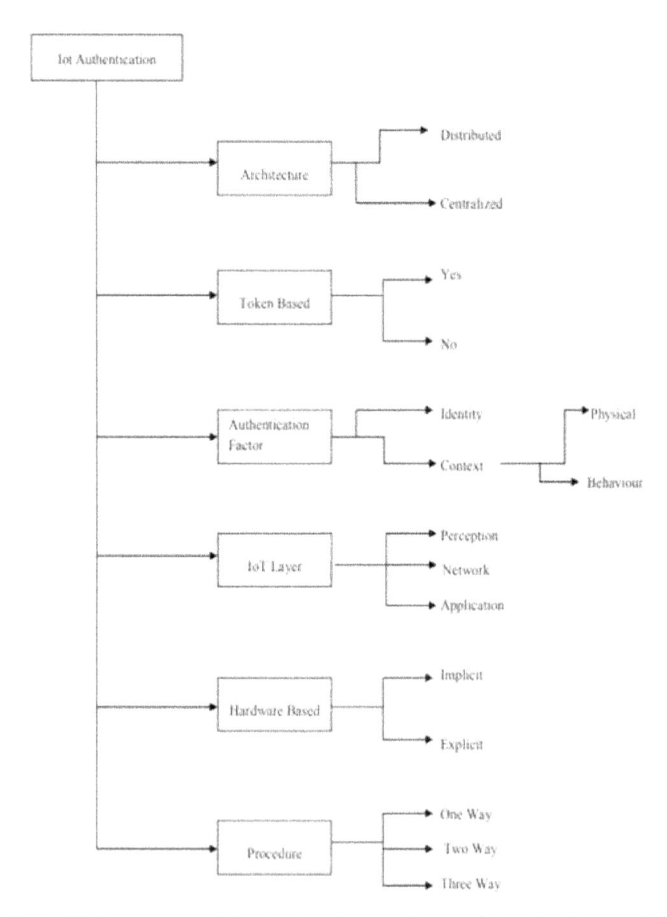

Fig. 2.17 Taxonomy of the Authentication Protocols in Health care IoT

Table 2.4 Security Services of the three layers in Health care IoT Architecture

IoT Layer	Security Services
Application Layer	Information Security Management
	Privacy Protection
	Authentication
Network Layer	Intrusion Detection
	Key Management
	Authentication
	Routing Security
	Communication Security
Perception Layer	Data Confidentiality
	Key Agreement
	Authentication
	Light weight Encryption

2.6 Summary

This chapter discussed the authentication and authorization mechanisms in health care IoT. It mainly focused on the architectures of IoT in different fields and the advantages and disadvantages of different algorithms. The taxonomy for authentication protocols in health care IoT is developed.

Table 2.5 Advantages and Disadvantages of Authentication algorithms Health care IoT

Ref	IoT layer	Hardware	Architecture	Identity context Credentials	Advantages	Disadvantages
Manyika etal.,(2015)	Application	Implicit	Centralized /Hierarchical	Encryption	Encapsulation Mechanism	
Kothmayr et al.,(2013)	Application and Network	Implicit	Centralized /Hierarchical	Encryption /RSA	Low overhead and High Inter-operability	Unreliable
Hammi etal.,(2017)	Perception	Implicit	Centralized /Hierarchical	Encryption /Asymmetric OTP	Resistance Against the Re-play Attacks and DoS attacks	Not Considered Performance Analysis
Du etal.,(2005)	Network	Implicit	Distributed / Hi-erarchical	Encryption /Sym-metric	Resistance Against the Node Capture Attack	Not considered the Energy Factor
Liu etal.,(2005)	Network	Implicit	Distributed / Hi-erarchical	Encryption /Sym-metric	Low over head and resistance against the Node Capture Attack	Not considered the location Privacy
Pranata etal.,(2012)	Application and Network	Implicit	Distributed / Hi-erarchical	Encryption /Asymmetric	Resistance against the mali-cious activities	Not Considered Performance Analysis
Hong etal.,(2013)	Application and Network	Implicit	Centralized /Hierarchical	Encryption /Asymmetric	No compatibility issues	Not Considered Performance Analysis
Wu etal.,(2011)	Application , Network and Perception	Implicit	Centralized /Flat	Encryption /Sym-metric	Provides Data Confidential-ity,Access Control,Client Privacy and Re-sistance Against the Attacks	-
Turkanov et al.,(2014)	Network and Per-ception	Implicit	Centralized /Flat	Encryption /Sym-metric	Authentication with RFID Tags	Not considered the location Privacy
Lee etal., (2014)	Network and Per-ception	Explicit	Centralized /Hierarchical	Encryption /Sym-metric Hash	Resistance against the Re-play, Man in the middle,breach attacks and stolen smart card attacks	Not concentrated the communica-tion cost
Ye etal., (2014)	Network and Per-ception	Implicit	Centralized /Hierarchical	Encryption /Asymmetric ECC	Resistance against the Re-play, DoS, Eaves dropping and MITM	Not discussed the attribute-based access control
Schmitt etal.,(2016)	Application, Net-work an Percep-tion	Implicit	Centralized/Flat	Encryption/ Asymmetric ECC+RSA	Resistance against the MITM attack	Not considered the Replay and DoS attacks
Porambage et al.,(2014)	Application, Net-work and Percep-tion	Implicit	Centralized /Dis-tributed	Encryption /Asymmetric ECC	Resistance against the DoS attacks	No resistance against the Node capture Attacks
Merkle etal., (1997)	Application	Implicit	Centralized /Hierarchical	Not Applicable	Resistance against Replay Attacks	Not Considered Performance Analysis
Chae etal., (2015)	Application	Implicit	Centralized /Flat	Encryption /AES	Cryptography and authentica-tion servers are maintained	Not Considered Performance Analysis
Bamasag et al.,(2015)	Application	Explicit	Distributed /Flat	No Encryption	Resistance again-stthe inside at-tacks and at client side second tier authentication is performed	There is no possi-bility of changing the credentials on both sides.

CHAPTER 3

SECURE DATA TRANSMISSION FOR PROTECTING USER PRIVACY IN MEDICAL INTERNET OF THINGS (M-IOT)

3.1 Introduction

In recent years, the developments in smart technologies are growing rapidly. Researchers have proposed many IoT applications such as health care management, transportation, smart home developments and logistics. In the future, IoT will be one field that will create a world where people and things can be integrated with communication networks to provide intelligent and autonomous services to human life. IoT is configured with sensors, actuators and mobile nodes for sensing the environments. IoT is also configured with a network layer for efficient data transmission between heterogeneous networks. Internet of Things (IoT) integrates heterogeneous devices together irrespective of their geographical location and capability. Hence, validating the users and granting access privileges to them are the most challenging security services. There are multiple authentication and authorization mechanisms proposed to address these concerns. Few proposals are complex and increase the resource consumption while others have their own pits and falls, encompassed in the literature survey.
Gaoetal.,(2012) addressed are al-time monitoring system for the cardiac function that can measure the heart rate of the patients and send data to the medical centers for better treatment through wireless technology or Bluetooth. Zhang et al.,(2012) proposed the method for medical data gathering by remote sleep monitoring that helps the doctors to analyze the patients condition during their sleep.Wanetal.,s healthcare (Wan et al., 2013; Ma et al., 2015;Hassan et al., 2017). (Zhang et al.,2017;Chenetal., 2015) proposed smart health care applications using the IoT.
In medical IoT, large volumes of heterogeneous medical data are gathered and this data contains information about the users.Therefore, user privacy is very important, once the medical data is tampered with or lost; it is very difficult to handle the privacy leakages. In the present era, how to ensure the security of medical data is always a research issue. Mni et al., (2013) proposed medical development with the help of information technology. They studied several key technologies and presented different methods for presenting the medical data from generation to storage. Jing etal., (2014) and Chen et

al., (2015) also studied different methods for securing the data in wireless networks. This chapter considers the security of data in the medical Internet of Things. The data are uploaded between the medical sensor nodes and the servers whereas download depends on the data transmission between the terminals and the servers. There is no specific method for preserving security in medical IoT. To secure the data in upload and download processes, a mechanism has been proposed to ensure secure data transmission across the devices used in medical IoT.
The objective of this proposal is to understand the mechanisms in authentication and authorization with respect to privacy and security in health care environment and to develop the authentication mechanism for securing the user privacy in medical IoT.

- To deliver mutual authentication solution and thereby minimize the number of messages to be exchanged.
- Make it lightweight by adopting simple operations in order to minimize the consumption of resources in the network.

This chapter puts forward a secure data transmission mechanism for M-IoT. It contains authentication, symmetric key generation and disjoint multipath data transmission modules.

- Authentication module validates the gateways with the cloud data servers and authorize the services mutually.
- Symmetric key generation module generates the key for encryption and decryption processes that reduces the processing complexity.
- The multipath data transmission module divides the encrypted data in to fragments that enable quick delivery and reduces the packet loss. Thereby the number of packet retransmission has been reduced and resource consumption also condensed.

The rest of the chapter is organized as follows: Section 3.2 deals with theliterature survey regarding the security mechanism applied to data protection in IoT. Section 3.3 deals with the architecture of the medical IoT. Section 3.4 presents the secure data transmission model in medical IoT. Section 3.5 explains the experimental results and finally, section 3.6 concludes the research work.

3.2 Literature survey

In recent years, IoT has gained popularity drastically. Many researchers have contributed their research in IoT with different proposals, but security is still a major concern to deal with in IoT. Encryption is a common method applied to preserve privacy. The common encryption techniques are AES, DES and RSA used for information systems as well as for medical IoT. Ning and Xu (2010) considered different security factors for IoT and also they managed to balance the tradeoff between business needs and privacy strength. For instance, to modify the privacy policies based on the business needs and also it needs to preserve the users privacy.

Lamport et al. (2010) proposed a technique to preserve privacy. It utilized the hash function pivoted authentication. But, the computation time of the model is high.Ding et al., (2009) suggested the hash pivoted encryption to protect data.Wuetal.,(2011) brought forth an algorithm with the light weight cryptographic one to protect data in the IoT.Added to that, they developed an ONS query mechanism to search the data in the applications of IoT. Song et al., (2011) proposed a method to transmit the data securely in IoT. They utilized a cooperative algorithm to successfully transmit data. Xie et al.,(2013) also proposed a scheme to transmit data securely in the IoT. In such a technique the trusted third party is adopted. But two parties alone will be authenticated. The technique of this kind of scheme is not acceptable where web applications have complexity.

In M-IoT, the data are mostly transmitted through the wireless medium and can be easily captured by intruders. Du etal.,(2003) proposed a key sharing method for wireless sensor networks (WSNs). The major drawback of this method is that the nodes share the same communication key. Hence the security is not guaranteed in this mechanism. Some schemes perform authentication before data transmission as suggested by Wang etal.,(2008) who proposed a two-way authentication based on an end-to-end encryption mechanism. This method involve third parties and it is defenseless to man-in-the-middle attacks.

Atzori et al., (2012) made a mention about the RFID reader can scan customers' RFID tags unnoticed by them. An unauthorized intruder could access customers information.Such an act can be easily done during the transmitting of information from the local server towards the remote server. In IoT,mostly the network that communicates utilizes small sensors by count. Apart from that, algorithms with light weight encryptions are utilized for encrypting the data (Medaglia and Serbanati,2009). Groce et al., (2010) proposed a protocol for security that works well in a generalized model, but it does not suit the medical-IoT applications. Forsstrom etal.,(2012) surveyed on security issues of IoT with respect to different heterogeneous networks and they managed to develop the distributed verification method for user authentication. However, this method is not suitable to deal with real-time dynamic data.

3.3 IoT Architecture

Figure 3.1 shows the common architecture of IoT applications. In general, the IoT architecture has four layers: sensing layer, data transmission layer, integration layer and application layer respectively. The communication model is shown in figure 3.2, for telemedicine with IoT where all medical data are gathered from sensor nodes. For instance, sensors like blood pressure sensors, RFID readers, blood-oxygen sensors and heart rate sensors are deployed in homes, hospitals, community public areas and health centers. These sensors use the mesh network to work in the Zig Bee transmission mode. If any user has to access the personal data, the identity of the user is authenticated by an RFID reader and the medical data is gathered by the sensor nodes.The gathered data are forwarded to the mesh node by the sensor nodes.The mesh node encapsulates the gathered data along with security processing and sends them to the nearest gateway.The gateway sends the medical data to the cloud data centers.The overall communication link is managed with mesh nodes, gateways, routers, and cloud data centers through the wireless mode. Finally the application layer provides the requested data to the users through PCs or mobiles. The data communication in the IoT is established with a variety of modes such as sensors in the deployed area communicating with a self-organized network and the gateways using the internet.

3.4 Proposed Secure DataTransmission Model

Most of the attacks and threats against devices and data security in IoT have a destructible effect because of their wireless radio access and connectivity to the Internet. The following module explains the procedure of securing data transmission in the Medical Internet of Things.

3.4.1 Network Initialization

In general, the sensor data transmission is done via a wireless medium. It is more vulnerable to attackers.The common attacks performed by the attackers are data leaking and malfunctioning. A secure data transmission method for medical-IoT which addresses the network initialization by managing the two-way authentication for registering the gateways at the servers is proposed. The proposed secure data transmission is explained as follows and the complete network initialization process of M-IoT is given in figure 3.3.

a) Networking in IoT:

IoT is composed of sensor nodes $\{L_1, L_2 ...... L_n\}$ as well as with sink nodes $\{N_1, N_2 ...... N_m\}$ and they are communicated with ZigBee wireless sensor networks W. The sensor nodes

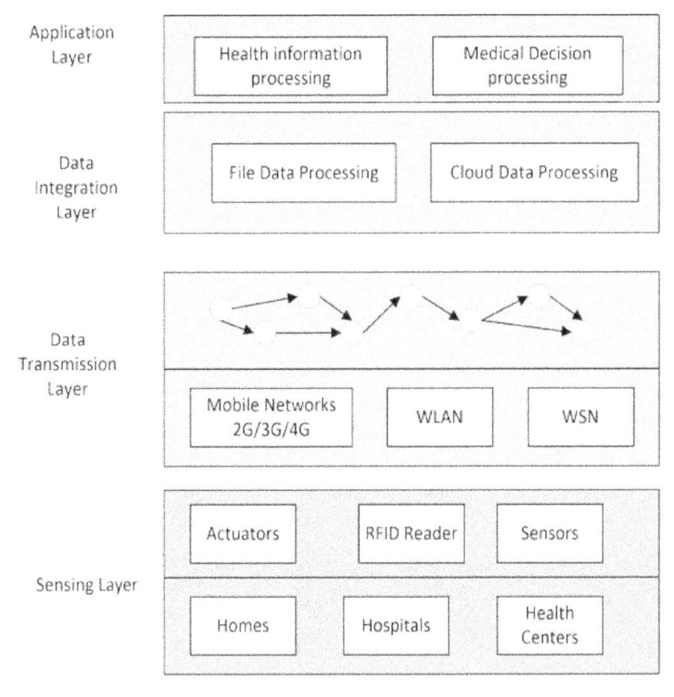

Fig. 3.1 Conventional Layered Architecture of Telemedicine through IoT

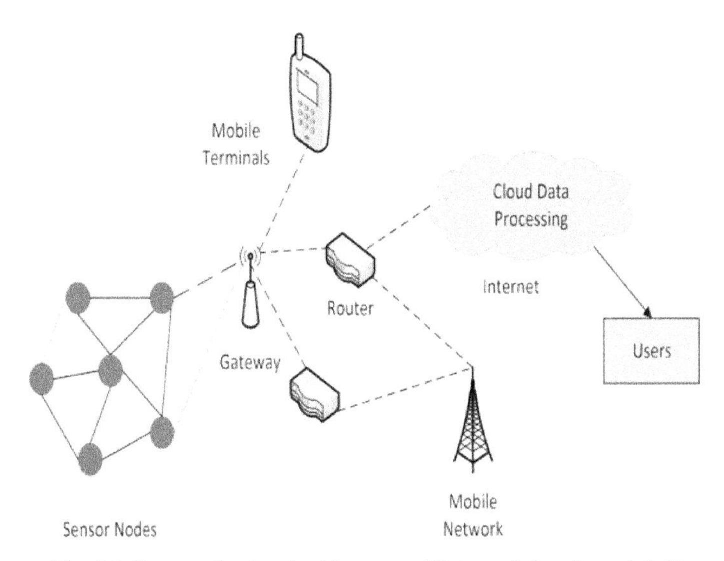

Fig. 3.2 Communication Architecture of Telemedicine through IoT

Gateway (G): Request made for Authentication(RQ_k)
Server (k): Verifies G
Gateway (G):$\{RQ_G, I_G, S_{k-G}, (H(\beta_G), RQk\} Server(k) : \{S_{k-G}(RQ_k, RQ_G, I_G\}$

are connected to the sink nodes and the sink nodes transfer the data through the gateway G to the internet.

b) Registration of Nodes:

When gateway G registers with the server K, G sends the password hashvalue β_G to

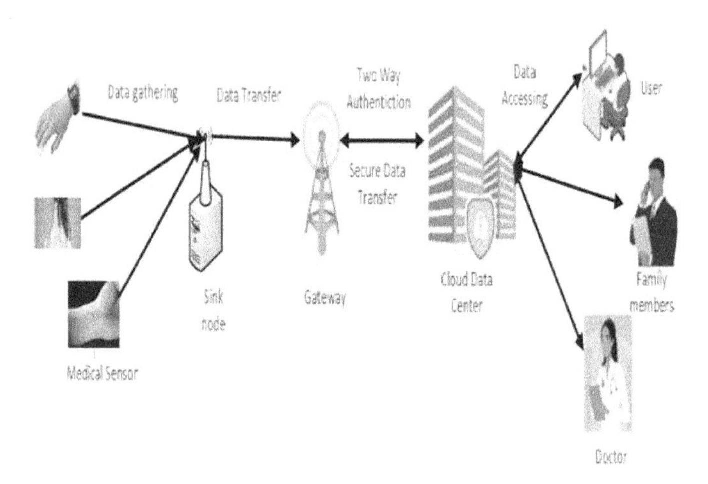

Fig. 3.3 Flow diagram for secure data transmission in M-IoT

the server K and then server K checks the received password with the password dictionary for authentication. All the gateway node passwords are registered in the dictionary. Figure 3.4 shows the registration procedure of the gateway nodes within the server.

c) Two-way authentication:

To preserve the security of the medical data, the authentication has to be performed between the gateway nodes G and the server K. In the proposed model, we are using the two-way authentication mechanismis used as shown below:

From the above notations, RQ_G and RQ_k indicate the requests for authentication made by a random number of gateways and servers. S_{k-G} represents the symmetric key representation for gateways and servers, $H(\beta_G)$ represents the password hash value for gateway and I_G represents the identity of the gateway node.

d) Symmetric Key Representation

Server K and gateway G generate the symmetric key S_{k-G} based on the symmetric

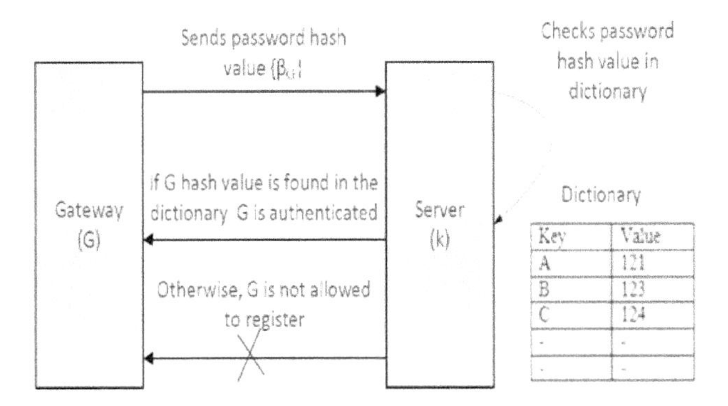

Fig. 3.4 Registrations of Gateway Nodes within the Server

key generation algorithm (Merkle, Ralph C, 1978). Both of them securely store the symmetric key S_{k-G} for encryption and decryption of medical data at the time of data transmission.

After completion of the two-way authentication mechanism between the servers and the gateways, they need to generate the symmetric key. This will be performed only when the gateway is initialized again. Algorithm 3.1 shows the symmetric key generation procedure for both the servers and the gateways.

e) Multipath DataTransmission

As per the above process, server K and gateway G completed the two-way authentication and share the common symmetric key S_{G-k} . To secure the data transmission more, the gateway G encrypts the data and it divides the cipher text into sub-parts for transferring them into multiple paths. This mechanism involves two sub-modules: one is the encryption of the collected data and the other one is the cipher text transmission.The complete procedure is shown in Figure 3.5.

3.4.2 Encryption

Consider the medicaldata of client D which contain different types of data, and sensing of these data are done by the sensors like $\{L_1, L_2 ..... L_n\}$ and it is transmitted to the sink node N_j. The representation of medical data D is given as follows:

$$D = \sum_{i=1}^{m} \{type\,(L_i) \oplus value\,(L_i)\} \quad (3.5)$$

After encrypting, the medical data D uses Advanced encryption Standard (AES-128) with symmetric key S, which is a shared key among all sensor nodes, sink nodes and gateways within the ZigBee region. The ciphertext μ after the encryption is given

Algorithm 3.1: Symmetric key generation (Merkle, Ralph C, 1978)

Input: P -> Large prime number selected by G and K,
δ -> generator selected from multiplicative group Z^*
Output: Symmetric Key
Begin
Step 1: Gateway G selects the integer x where $\{1 \le x \le P-2\}$
Step 2: G computes the X and sends it to the server K

$$X = \delta^x \bmod P \qquad (3.1)$$

Step 3: Server K selects the integer y where $\{1 \le y \le P-2\}$
Step 4: K computes the Y and sends it to the Gateway G

$$Y = \delta^y \bmod P \qquad (3.2)$$

Step 5: G computes the symmetric key S_G and generates the random number RQ_G and sends the encrypted data {E (RQ_G), RQ_G} to Server K.

$$S_G = Y^x \bmod P \qquad (3.3)$$

Step 6: Server S computes the symmetric key S_k and generates the random numberRQ_k and sends the encrypted data {E(RQ_k) , RQ_k, RQ_G} to Server K.

$$S_k = X^y \bmod P \qquad (3.4)$$

Step 7: Gateway G receives and decrypts the {E(RQ_k) , RQ_k, RQ_G} and replies true to the server. G and K commonly share the symmetric key $S_{G\text{-}k}$ for completing the key sharing process.

End

as follows:

$$\mu = E_{s(D)} \qquad (3.6)$$

For instance, the cipher text μ of the medical data in node N1 is sent to the neighboring nodes and these nodes transmit the cipher text μ to the gateways G. After the symmetric key is received, the gateways decrypt the cipher text and retrieve the plain text.

$$D = dec_s(\mu) \qquad (3.7)$$

3.4.3 Disjoint Ciphertext

The cipher text is divided into several sub-parts $\{\mu 1, \mu 2, ... \mu n\}$ by gateway G for each sub-part . The gateway G adds a sequence number and identification number ID

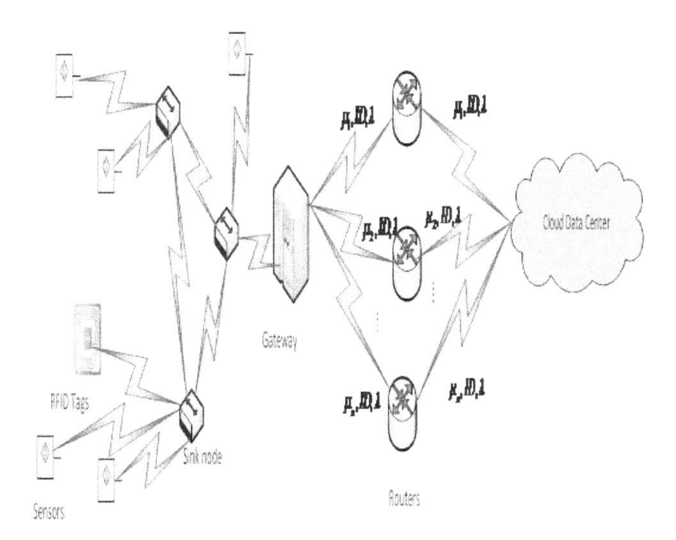

Fig. 3.5 Multipath data transmission in M-IoT

and the message format is given as follows:

$$d_i = \{\mu, ID, \lambda\} \tag{3.8}$$

The id validity is verified by the server K using the hash function H(x), and gateway G calculates the authentication code using the secret key

$$h = H_{S_{K-G}}(\mu, ID, \lambda, h) \tag{3.9}$$

In the next step, the gateway G sends the message on the selected path which is given as:

$$PT_I = (\mu, ID, \lambda, h) \tag{3.10}$$

After collecting all the subparts of the cipher text with the same sequence number of the same gateway G, then server K will recognize the cipher text as:

$$\mu = \sum_{i=1}^{n} \mu_i \tag{3.11}$$

Finally, server K performs the decryption operation to the collected cipher text as:

$$D = dec_{S_{K-G}}(\mu) \tag{3.12}$$

3.5 Experimental Results

The Contiki operating system is a C-based OS designed for embedded systems lightweight which is capable of multitasking. It is highly memory efficient and open-sourced, allowing custom modifications and improvements from a wide community. It has dynamic applications of loading and unloading capabilities for services and applications. This gives it numerous advantages in terms of resource utilization and allows a highly efficient kernel driven architecture for sensor networks. This makes it an ideal operating system for the implementation of secure authentication using symmetric cryptography techniques. The proposed model is implemented in the Contiki environment using the Java programming language. In order to implement the device registration phase of the protocol, cryptographic provider libraries such as Flexi provider and bouncy castle are used. Similarly, to implement the authentication phase of the protocol, the AES protocol implementation, available in the bouncy castle library, is used. It is then simulated in the Cooja simulator under the Contiki OS environment. It should be noted that the collected data are captured from the corresponding devices that are provided and used by an anonymized patient of Bio Assists platform (https://bioassist.gr/, accessed on 22 June 2019).

3.5.1 Security Analysis

For securing data transmission in M-IoT, it has to deal with wireless sensor networks, symmetric key generation and disjoint multipath transmission. The security analysis against each of these components is explained in the following subsections.

3.5.1.1 Wireless Sensor Network Security

In WSNs, the ZigBee protocol defines the security for the MAC layer, Network layer and Application Layer. It also manages the security by providing the symmetric key generation. AES-128 is the encryption technique used to generate the key and it is open to all the devices. Each device has to access the algorithm and the key must be the same.

Security through Authentication: Gateway G has to authenticate with Server S before the data transmission takes place. If the two-way authentication mechanism is not successful between the G and S, then the server S refuses the gateway and marks it as a fake gateway. Therefore, it is very important to validate the authentication of gateways and servers. Table 3.2 shows the analysis of authentication security. The proposed protocol uses two-way authentication for managing the gateways and also it has the ad-

Table 3.1 Comparison of AES Versions

Parameters	AES-128	AES-192	AES-256
Data Block Size	128	192	256
Matrix Block	4*4	4*6	4*8
Number of Round	10	12	14

vantage of the hash function. The proposed protocol is more secure than the existing protocols (Hwang and Yeh,2002;Wang etal.,2008). Hwang and Yehs protocol does not contain the gateway node verification method.

Replay Attacks: Intercepting a message for replay attacks on the proposed system is impossible. After receiving a login request, the system verifies whether the timestamp is within the legal delay; if not the system denies the request.

DoS Attacks: In the proposed model, the gateways need to be registered under the servers before the data transmission. Therefore, the servers validate the authenticity of the gateways and it avoids the Denial of Service attacks.

Server and Gateway Forging: The proposed model follows two-way authentication mechansism between the server and the gateways. Therefore, both the server and the gateways need to be authenticated. Hence, forging of gateways and server is not possible.

Hash Function: The proposed model uses AES encryption protocol for data encryption. This AES encryption process takes the help of hash function to generate the cipher text.

Public key method: The proposed model does not use the public key mechansism for data access. It uses the symmetric key cryptograpy for data access.

Table 3.2 Analysis of Authentication Protocols

Security	**Wang etal.,(2008)**	**Hwang and Yeh (2002)**	**Proposed Method**
Preventing Replay attacks	Yes	No	Yes
Preventing DoS attacks	No	No	Yes
Preventing Server Forging	Yes	Yes	Yes
Hash function	No	Yes	Yes
No public key method	Yes	Yes	Yes
Preventing gateway Forging	Yes	Yes	Yes

3.5.1.2 Symmetric key generation security

The symmetric key generation is the process of managing the security using the three-way handshake process. This will prevent the intruders to gain access to the medicaldata which are in transit. The proposed protocol generates the symmetric key for encryption and decryption of the medical data. Table3.3 shows the analysis of the existing mechanisms with the proposed approach. The proposed approach has the advantage of a three-way hand shake when compared to the Diffie-Hellman (Bressonetal., 2002; Xieet al., 2013).

Table 3.3 Analysis of key generation Mechanisms

Security	Diffie-Hellman (2002)	Xieetal.,(2013)	Proposed Method
Preventing Integrity Attacks	Yes	No	Yes
Preventing Known key attacks	Yes	No	Yes
Preventing wiretap attacking	Yes	Yes	Yes
Three-way handshake	No	No	Yes

3.5.1.3 Multipath Data Transmission Security

The multipath data transmission mechanism is more secure and it is very difficult for the attackers to gain access to the medical data compared to the single path data transmission. In the proposed method, the security is provided in two modules: one is the data which have been encrypted and the other is the encrypted data which have been divided in to different fragments to avoid the Man in the Middle attacks and to gain access to the complete data.

The performance of the algorithms is tested with the NS2 simulator (Issariyakul and Hossain, 2011). Inorder to facilitate the test, the data partition of size 126 bits has been considered in the disjoint multipath data transmission. In this method, only the sink node has the responsibility to collect the medical data from the medical sensor nodes and the collected data is sent to the server. The position of the route nodes and the sink nodes are fixed in the network. Algorithms proposed by Hwang and Yeh (2002)Diffie-Hellman Bresson et al., (2002) and Xie et al., (2013) produced larger delays compared to the proposed algorithm. The proposed algorithm uses symmetric key encryption which also introduces some delay but it is acceptable in real time. The transmission delay of the algorithms will increase further if the medical data are gathered from different regions. Figure 3.6 shows the comparison of delay with respect to the number of partitions.

Table 3.4 examines the comparison of delay with respect to the number ofpartitions.

Table 3.4 Number of Partitions versus Delay

Number of Partitions	Delay (ns)			
	Proposed Algorithm	Xie et al	Diffie Hellman	Hwang and yeh
2	4	18	19	21
4	5	25	27	28
6	6	29	35	36
8	9	36	40	42
10	10	42	50	53
12	12	64	66	68
14	14	57	58	60
16	5	66	67	68
18	16	68	69	72

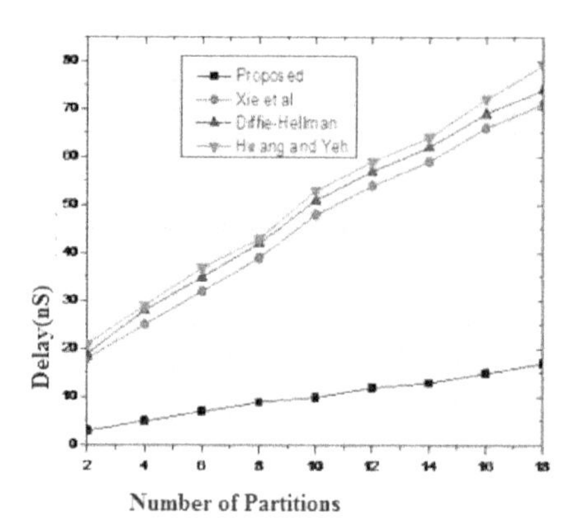

Fig. 3.6 Comparison of Delay with respect to the Number of Partitions

The performance of the proposed algorithm is also tested with the downloaded data.The users of different types of data can access the data such as querying, updating and deleting. At the same time, it provides security to the users and also increases the response time to access the data from the server. In this experiment, the access controls in terms of users and the type of data and diagnostic data are divided. Figure 3.7 shows that the response time is very large when the users are increased drastically.This is not suitable for real-time applications.Therefore, authentication management has to be simplified based on the frequent accessing users.

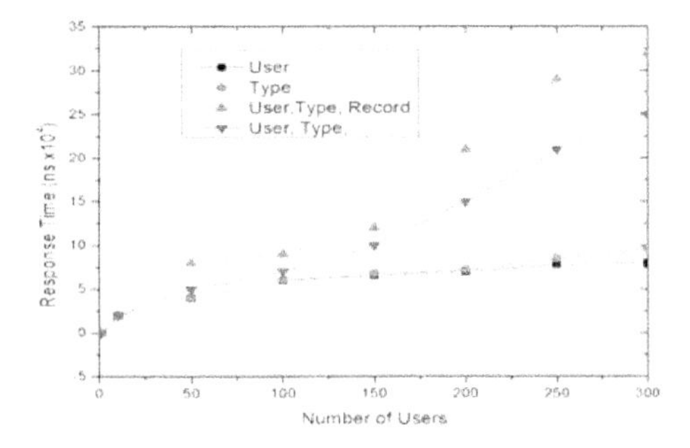

Fig. 3.7 Comparison of Response Time with respect to Number of Users

Figures 3.8 and 3.9 show the average data transfer rate of the proposed method with encryption in the ZigBee network. It is observed that the data transfer rate of the proposed method is maximum due to the encryption but it is better at the point of security compared to Hwang and Yeh (2013), Bresson et al. (2002) and Xie (2013) methods. The proposed method uses the AES-128 algorithm to encrypt the data and also manages the multipath data transmission approach to increase the data transmission rate.

Table 3.5 examines the comparison of Average Number of bits transferred without Encryption.

Table 3.5 Average Number of bits transferred without Encryption

Simulation Time	Number of Bits			
	Proposed Algorithm	Diffie Hellman	Xie et al	Hwang and yeh
200	50	100	83	80
300	72	110	108	83
400	88	128	118	110
500	92	150	131	128
600	108	155	134	132

Table 3.6 examines the comparison of Average Number of bits transferred with Encryption.

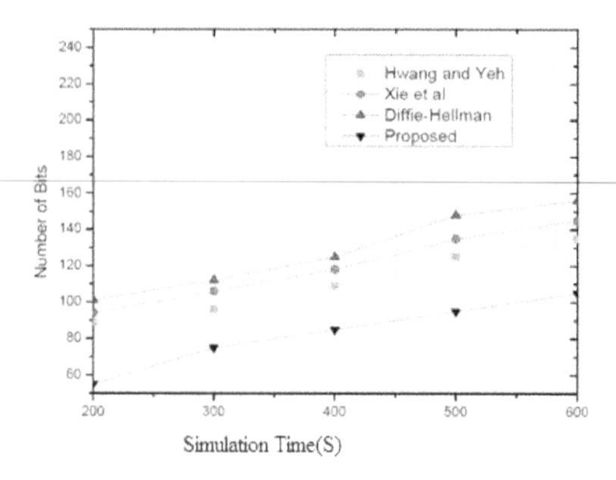

Fig. 3.8 Average number of bits transferred without encryption

Table 3.6 Average Number of bits transferred with Encryption

Simulation Time	Number of Bits			
	Proposed Algorithm	Diffie Hellman	Xie et al	Hwang and yeh
200	88	120	139	158
300	92	129	143	162
400	95	132	150	171
500	108	138	158	189
600	110	142	170	192

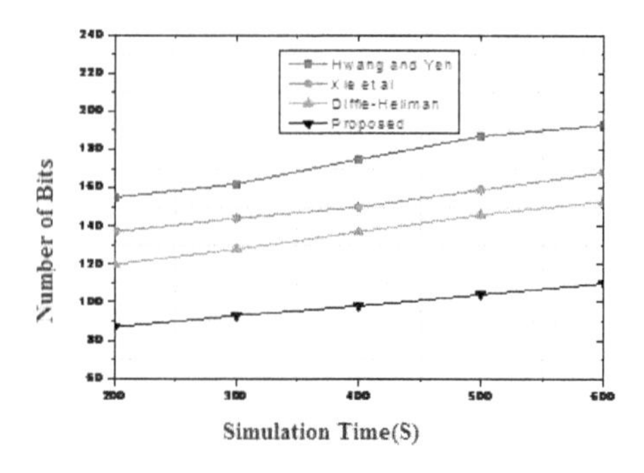

Fig. 3.9 Average number of bits transferred with encryption

Figure 3.10 shows the comparison of legitimate users granted access. It is observed that the number of legitimate users who were granted access is higher when compared to other existing algorithms.Therefore the proposed approach has better performance compared to the other algorithms.
Table 3.7 examines the Average Number of Legitimate Users granted to Access the data.

Table 3.7 Average Number of Legitimate Users granted to Access the data

Number of Users	Number of Legitimate Users			
	Proposed Algorithm	**Hwang and yeh**	**Xie et al**	**Diffie Hellman**
100	59	50	59	32
150	88	62	70	48
200	92	89	72	52
250	128	102	90	68
300	151	129	92	72
350	170	132	110	88

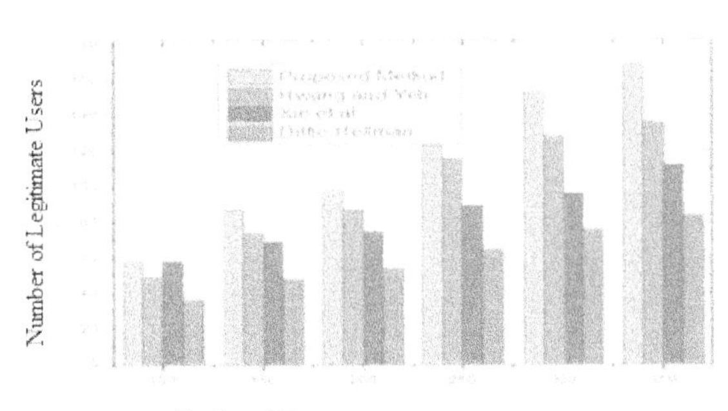

Fig. 3.10 Average Number of Legitimate Users granted to Access the data

3.6 Summary

This chapter discussed about the model for secure data transmission in Medical-IoT. The proposed model considers three modules such as Two-way authentication, symmetric key generation and disjoint multipath data transmission. The enhanced symmetric key encryption mechanism by managing the three-way hand shake between the gateways and cloud servers is developed. The disjoint multipath data transmission provides high security by fragmenting the encrypted data so that attackers cannot obtain data residing in the server. Secure access to the server is obtained through authentication and authorized access. The experimental analysis evidenced proof that the algorithm in the proposal is capable of authentication and also decreases the delay for data transmission.

CHAPTER 4

HYBRID ENCRYPTION MODEL FOR MANAGING DATA SECURITY IN MEDICAL INTERNET OF THINGS

4.1 Introduction

In recent years, IoT is treated as one of the emerging technologies which connect sensors, smart mobiles and smart infrastructure through the internet.The sensor devices communicate through wireless or wired medium to exchange the data. The IoT environment can connect things at anytime from anywhere and it also provides any type of service (Palattella et al., 2013; Chiuchisan et al., 2015).The utilization of IoT is extensively applied in different areas such as smart vehicles, smart homes, smart environment monitoring and smart cities.Medical/Healthcare data are the most sensitive and critical data type. Inversion of single bit could cause a wrong diagnosis and become a life threat. Simple symmetric key algorithms can offer effective data protection in the field of IoT and efficient medical data management.Huge volume of medical data are stored in the cloud servers and those servers are vulnerable to tampering (active attack) and eavesdropping (passive attack). Again data sharing through M-IoT leads to some serious issues of security and privacy.
The management of e-health records in the field of MedicalIoT (M-IoT) leads to the improvement of quality and security to patients care and it also improves the healthcare services by reducing the cost and time (Whitmor et al., 2015; Yang, 2015). The M-IoT provides great opportunities to transform the health care system. The M-IoT has the ability to connect different sensor devices and it enables remote monitoring of patients, elderly care and rehabilitation of patients. M-IoT also reduces medical costs and improves the quality of health care.
The sharing of data through M-IoT leads to some serious issues of security and privacy. Huge volumes of medical data are stored in the cloud servers and those servers are vulnerable to tampering and eaves dropping attacks (Hassanalieragh et al.,2015; Pilkington, 2017). The major issue faced by M-IoT is the security of medical data without minimizing the data re-usability (Singhetal.,2015). In M-IoT remote access control is one of the crucial mechanisms to restrict a third party from accessing medical data. To secure data confidentiality, the medical data is converted in to an encrypted format and

uploaded to the cloud for storage (Rajeevetal.,2016). Attribute-Based encryption (ABE) is the general approach used for encrypting sensor data, but it is not suitable for the M-IoT data due to the complexity of computations. IoT usually has small sensor devices that are limited to energy and computation capacity (Thotaetal.,2018).Therefore it is required to design an efficient and low complex mechanism for encrypting the medical data (Elhoseny et al.,2018; Raju, and Saritha, 2016).

This chapter concentrates on developing the architecture for medical data management in IoT. This architecture will provide secure communication for datasharing among doctors and patients in normal and emergency conditions.This proposal focuses on developing an authentication Model which can store huge volumes of data collected by sensor nodes and to propose a security mechanism to preserve Data confidentiality, Data Integrity and Access control.

- To design an authentication protocol for resource-constrained sensor networks, which are the underlying technology of Internet of Things applications.

- To evaluate the resistance of the model developed against the known active and passive attacks in the perception layer of IoT.

This chapter proposes an architecture for managing the large volumes of medical data generated by the sensor nodes. This architecture provides a secure communication for data sharing among doctors and patients in normal and emergency conditions.

- An efficient access control mechanism is developed by combining symmetric cryptography and attribute-based encryption.

- This hybrid algorithm reduced the computation overhead at the time of the encryption and decryption process. The proposed model is resistant against Replay attack, Man-in-the middle attack and Impersonation attack.

The rest of the chapter is organized as follows: Section 4.2 deals with related work. Section 4.3 develops the architecture for data management in IoT. Section4.4 narrates the security of the model for M-IoT. Section 4.5 explains the simulation results. Finally, section 4.6 concludes the research work.

4.2 Literature Survey

IoT is treated as an evolutionary paradigm to communicate thing-to-human, thing-to-thing, and human-to-thing (Singh etal.,2014). The security in the field of IoT attracted more researchers from both industries and academics to manage the services. The usage of encryption mechanisms in the field of IoT leads to security protection and efficient medical data management. Bernabe et al., (2016) developed light weight authentication schemes for medical IoT using hash-based message authentication to verify the integrity of data. Bae etal.,(2016) developed the ecliptic curve cryptography (ECC) which used a lightweight control mechanism for IoT. The major drawbacks of this model are poor generality, poor flexibility and poor scalability. Therefore, this model is not suitable for IoT applications (Khemissa Tandjaoui D, 2015; Yao et al., 2015).
Song et al., (2003) proposed searchable based encryption for text search in the encrypted data. This work gained more attention from the researchers to continue their research in the keyword search issues on the cipher text. Goh etal.,(2003) proposed the attribute-based encryption method which contained both the cipher text and secret key associated with the attributes set. The retrieving of a message is possible from the cipher text if the users key matches with the cipher text attributes.
Bethencourt and Amit (2007) mentioned that the RFID reader could scan customers RFID tags unnoticed by them. An unauthorized intruder can access customers information .Such an act can be easily done during the transmission of information from the local server to the remote server (Raju and Saritha, 2016). In IoT, the number of sensors i.e. the count of sensors,is managed for communication in the network. Apart from that, algorithms with light weight encryptions are utilized for encrypting the data (Groceand Katz, 2010).
Groce et al., (2007) proposed a protocol for security that works well in a generalized model, but it does not suit medical-IoT applications. This is because the IoT applications are connected with smart devices which require complex cryptographic mechanisms. Forsstrom et al., (2012) surveyed on the security issues of IoT with respect to different heterogeneous networks and they managed to develop the distributed verification method for user authentication. However, this method is not suitable for dealing with real-time dynamic data.
Even though authentication and authorization are essential to achieve confidentiality and therefore privacy, they may also harm a users privacy. For example, when communicating over the internet, it is almost always necessary to disclose information that can be used to identify devices, users, or natural persons, such as IP addresses of communicating parties. Messages sent or actions taken by entities may be linked to the same entity. That may make users vulnerable to undesired or malicious tracking (Krasnova, 2017).

But even when the communicating parties are successful in concealing these properties for third parties, privacy issues may occur as a result of authentication. This is because authentication generally consists of an identity (such as a user name), and a token (such as a password or a cryptographic proof). Therefore, there must always be a party that controls a database with identities. The entity that is responsible for maintaining this list of identities is therefore (at least technically) able to track users in a system, creating potential privacy problems (Krasnova, 2017).
Zhou et al. (2017) discusses how authentication can play a role in preserving users privacy. When identifying themselves, users may for example adopt a pseudonym rather than an identity, known as pseudonymization. A pseudonym may protect the users privacy because the pseudonym cannot be linked directly to the user. However, it may be necessary to update pseudonyms periodically, which can be hard (Zhou et al., 2017). Besides that, each pseudonym is unique which potentially makes entities identifiable if additional information is available. Another approach is by using group signatures, which are a form of digital signatures in which any member of a group can sign on behalf of the others. The identity of a member is therefore not necessarily disclosed (Khader, 2007).
However, because this signature is the same for an entire group, this may not allow for fine-grained access control which is often necessary in IoT scenarios. It is also possible to authenticate users via attributes, which are properties of users such as environmental conditions like time and locations (Alpr et al., 2016). Some argue that using attributes instead of identities for access control improves users privacy, because decisions for granting or denying access can be made solely on those qualities that are seen as essential (Alpr et al., 2016). Attribute-based authentication allows users to control their personal information, by data minimization, and limitation of goal (Krasnova, 2017).

4.3 Proposed Model

This section describes the model which enables the medical-IoT such as healthcare and hospitals to manage the sensor nodes for collecting the data. The proposed model is efficient in storing huge volumes of data collected by the sensor nodes. Since these data are highly confidential, a security method for preserving data integrity, data confidentiality and access control is developed.

To achieve the above-mentioned objectives, the architecture shown in Figure 4.1 is developed. The architecture comprises of three sets of users, patients health care professionals and general users. It contains the following modules:

Table 4.1 Nomenclature

PU_k	Publickey
RS_K	Randomly generated Symmetric Key
M_k	Master key
PR_k	Private Key
S_k	Secret key
A_P	Access privileges
U_{ID}	Represents User ID
H	Represents the Hash value
D	Represents the health data
M	Represents the medical data
ARP	Represents the read mode access privilege
ARW	Represents the write mode access privilege
(PS)W	Password for the file at write mode
(PS) CS_p	Password for the cloud

- Smart devices are the sensor nodes that monitor the patient's health condition and collect data at regular intervals.

- The health care professionals access the stored medical data using the monitoring applications.

- The Health care Authority (H_A) is responsible for the security policies of the hospitals or health care institutes.

- Cloud storage is used for storing medical data and also for preserving data security.

In the proposed architecture, each patient is attached to light weight sensor nodes. These sensor nodes enable continuous monitoring of patients and collect different data such as motions, heart beats and physiological signals. Each sensor node forwards the sensed data to the gateway where the data aggregation is performed along with the encryption using the randomly generated symmetric key (RS_K). The encrypted data are stored in the cloud. Doctors or health care professionals can use monitoring applications to supervise the health of patients from any location. The health care professionals can download the data from the cloud and decrypt it using the secret key. The monitoring applications use RS_K for medical data encryption and uses H_A for access privileges.

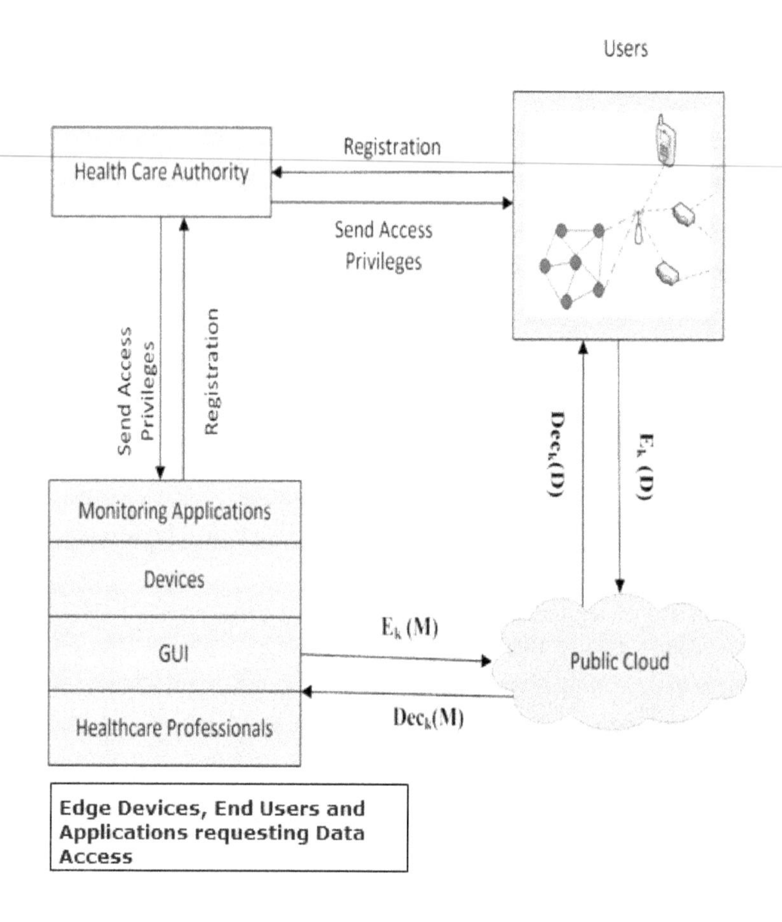

Fig. 4.1 Proposed Model for Medical IoT

4.4 Security Model for M-IoT

This section deals with the security model for the proposed method along with the provided services. The proposed security model has the following parts: users, healthcare authority and cloud. It is considered that the communication between the users, H_A and the cloud is secured by using SSL protocol. In communication, SSL provides data confidentiality and data integrity, but the data need to be encrypted at the user level to store the data in the cloud. The public key infra structure is used to maintain the public and private key pair of each party.

Algorithm4.1:Validating the New user

UserID:UId//UserID

UId→PKI: UId// PKI generates the public Key PUk and Private Key PRk

PKI→UID: Es{PUk, PRk}

UId →HA // HA uses the CP-ABE algorithm for generating the secret key Sk and Access policies AP to the user

HA→UId{Sk,AP}

AP:ARP// Readmode

HA→Csp// cloud adds UId along with its PUk to the user list (Lu).

4.4.1 Security Implementation

At the initial stage, the Healthcare Authority (H_A) attribute set uses an Attribute-Based Encryption (ABE) algorithm for generating the public key (PU_k) and the masterkey(M_k). The publickey (PU_k) is disclosed to all the users and it is used to encrypt and decrypt the data. The master key (M_k) is kept secret from the users. To disclose the PU_k, the H_A ciphers it with the private key (PR_k) and forwards it to the cloud service providers (Csp). The user downloads the PU_k and validates the authenticity.

4.4.2 Authenticating and Authorizing Health care Professionals

In Medical-IoT, users can join and leave the network at any time. If the a new user joins the network, the H_A has to assign the secret key (S_k) along with the access privileges to the new user. The access privileges (A_P) provide the flexibility to the new user to encrypt and decrypt the data before sending it to the cloud. Algorithm 4.1 shows the procedure of validating new users in the network.

As an initial step, the PKI generates PU_k, PR_k for the user, then H_A uses the CP-ABE algorithm for generating the S_k and A_P to the user. H_A requests the cloud to add the user UId to the user list (Lu). After receiving the request from the H_A the cloud adds U_{Id} along with its PU_k to the user list(Lu). Once the user gateway creates the communication with the H_A, then the user receives the S_k, A_P and PR_k.

Table 4.2 Comparison of MD5 and SHA-256 hash functions

Algorithm	**Output Size**	**Rounds**	**Security**	**Speed**
MD5	128 bits	64	Low	High
SHA-256	256 bits	24	High	Low

The security parameters of the health care professionals and the patients are different. The patients need to encrypt the health data before sending it into the cloud and it is in read-only mode. The medical data sent by the health care professionals need to be encrypted and it is in both read R and write W mode. H_A provides the access privileges of patients and healthcare professionals in different methods. The access privileges of healthcare professionals are composed of two parts: one is for encrypting the medical data and the other is for the protection of the write mode. Algorithm 4.1 shows the procedure of authenticating and authorizing health care professionals.

Algorithm 4.2:Authenticating and Authorizing Hp

HealthcareProfessionals:HP

HP→PKI: HP // PKI generates the public Key PUk and Private Key PRk
PKI→Hp:Es{PUk,PRk}
Hp→HA//HA uses CP-ABE algorithm for generating the secret key Sk and access policies AP to the Hp

HA→HP{Sk,AP}

AP:ARP+AWp//ReadandWritemode

HA→Csp//cloud adds Hp along with its PUk to the list.

4.4.3 Management of Health Data

The health data is collected by the sensor nodes and the data is accessed only in the read mode. The sensor nodes continuously send the sensed data to gateway G. The gateway G executes Algorithm 4.2 before it uploads the data to the cloud.

In Algorithm 4.3, U_{Id} forwards the health data to the gateway. The gateway G generates the RS_k using the symmetric key encryption algorithm, then computes the hash value using the SHA-256 algorithm. The SHA-256 algorithm is a widely used hash

function with a 256-bit hash value. This algorithm is more secure than the MD5 algorithm. The major advantages of SHA-256 over MD5 are given in Table 4.2.
G encrypts the D and H using the RS_k and adds the access privileges to the encrypted RSk and finally forwards the encrypted health data$U_{Id}, E_k RS_k, A_p, E_k(D+H)RS_k$ to the cloud service provider CSp.

Algorithm 4.3: Management of Health data

Health data:D
User ID: UID
Random symmetric Key: RSk
Hash value:H
Gateway: G
UID→D
G→Generate (RSk)//Gateway generates Random symmetric key RSk

G→Compute (H) // Gateway computes the hash value using the SHA-256 algorithm
RSk→Ek(D+H)//Encrypts the health data and hash value
Ap: ARP// Gateway adds access privileges

G→CSp{UId,Ek{RSk, Ap},Ek(D+H)RSk}//Gateway the encrypted health data to the cloud service provider CSp

After the gateway transmits the encrypted data to the CSp, the users can access the data and decrypt it by submitting the secret key S_k. The user has to perform the additional step of validating the RS_k with the CP-ABE algorithm.After decrypting,the user has to validate the data integrity. If any discrepancies are noticed in the decrypted data, the user has to send the message to the H_A.

4.4.4 Management of Medical Data

The medical data consist of prescriptions, diagnostics and reports generated by the health care professionals. This data can be modified by any other users who have the write access. Therefore, to restrict the write access, a password is provided for each file. If any user has to perform the write operation on the file, they need to submit the password of the specific file. Algorithm 4.4 shows the procedure of adding medical data by the health care professionals.
The health care professionals follow the same procedure for reading the medical datafrom the cloud which is followed for health data. But for write access, the health care pro-

fessional has to be validated to gain data access for modifications.

Algorithm 4.4: Management of Medical Data

Medical data: M
User ID: UID
Password: (PS)w
UID→M
G→Generate (RSk)//Gateway generates Random symmetric key RSk
 	
G→Compute(H)//Gateway computes the hash value using the SHA-256algorithm
 	
RSk→Ek(M+H) //Encrypts the medical data and hash value
 	
G→Ek{RSk,ARp}//Gateway encrypts the Random symmetric key RSk and access policy.
 	
G→Ek{PS,AWp} the health care professional has to submit the password (PS) of the file to the CSp
 	
Ap→ARP+AWP//Gateway adds access privileges
 	
G→$CS_p\{U_{Id},E_k\{RS_k,A_p\},(PS)_w,(PS)_{CSp},E_k(M+H)_{RSk}\}$//Gateway the encrypted health data to the cloud service provider CS_p

4.5 Performance Analysis

In M-IoT, the sensor nodes are deployed into different regions such as homes, public areas and hospitals. All sensor nodes gather information about the users medical data like blood pressure, heart rate, ECG, blood glucose levels at regular intervals. The collected data is forwarded to the sink nodes.The sink nodes combine the medical data and forward it to the gateway. The gateway splits the data into fragments. These fragments are transmitted through different routers and from them the fragments are transmitted to the cloud storage service.Further, doctors, patients, nurses, family members and managers can access the data from cloud storage with their specified user permissions. The symmetric key generation is carried out by using the AES-128 algorithm.
AES-128 uses 128-bit blocks which is efficient and secure and it takes less time to compute compared to the 192 and 256 bits keys. It takes 10 rounds to generate the symmetric key. It is stronger than the DES and 3DES algorithms. The comparison of encryption algorithms is given in Table 4.3.

Table 4.3 Comparison of AES, DES and 3DES Symmetric algorithms

Factors	DES	3DES	AES
KeySize	56 bits	68 and 112 bits	128,192 and 256 bits
Ciphertype	Symmetric	Symmetric	Symmetric
Crypt analysis	Weak substitutional tables,vulnerable to linear and differential attacks	Vulnerable to differential and brute force attacks	Strong against all the attacks
Security	Inadequate	Some weaknesses are still exists	Considered to be more secure
Rounds	16	48	10(128-bits),12(192- bits and 14(256-bits)

4.6 Security Analysis

The proposed model manages the data confidentiality, data integrity and data authenticity at the time of data transfer. It provides effective access control over the files stored in the cloud. Each medical file is encrypted using the symmetric key and CP-ABE is used for encrypting the symmetric key (Kallahalla et al., 2003). The CP-ABE algorithm is efficient against unauthorized access. From this, it is proven that arandom secret key ensures confidentiality and guarantees the security of the stored medical data. In this section, the ABE algorithm is compared with the proposed algorithm with different attribute sets and random access privileges for the medical data. For simulation, the ABE tool kit (Medaglia and Serbanati, 2009) and advanced encryption standard (ABE) of Open SSL for encryption are considered.

The proposed model resist against the following attacks:

Replay Attacks: During each handshaking session, the scrambled medical data conveyed in channels at one specific moment differs from that of another moment because the matrix M for encryption is randomly generated, and such an inconformity is unpredictable. Therefore, the attacker is unable to conduct a fake inquiry by replay attacks.

Man-in-the-Middle Attacks: The proposed scheme is resilient against man-in-the-middle attacks considering two concerns: the first is the attack during communication between entities of the system that requires verifying if the public key is correct and belongs to the person or entity claimed, and has not been tampered with or replaced by a malicious third party; the second is ensuring that the Public Key of CP-ABE system is the original P_K which is provided by the concerned healthcare authority. In the proposed scheme, to respond to the first issue, each emitter has to send a digital certificate specifically issued by the research studys public key infrastructure to the receiver. Then, the receiver verifies the validity of the certificate by using the public key of PKI provided for this study. For the second issue, the CP-ABE P_K is signed by the Healthcare authority, and any entity of the system can verify the authenticity of CP-ABE public key to use it.

Impersonation Attack: An impersonation attack occurs when an attacker poses as a legitimate party in order to access sensitive information. If an attacker can impersonate a legitimate user, then they can forge a message to appear as if it was sent by the patient.Even if the attacker knows the patients public key, they still cannot forge messages since it is signed with the patients private key.

Figure 4.2 and Figure 4.3 show the performance analysis of the encryption and decryption process in both ABE and the proposed algorithms. For this, the overhead of the computation and a different set of attributes (i.e.,access policies) are compared. From Figures 4.2 and 4.3, it is observed that the proposed algorithm is efficient in reducing the computation overhead compared to the ABE algorithm. The proposed algorithm has an efficient access mechanism with respect to encryption and decryption operations.The proposed method uses the AES algorithm for encrypting the medical data and for encrypting the AES key it uses the CP-ABE algorithm. It is noted that the proposed algorithm reduced the overhead by about 15% to 21%in encryption, and by 35% to 45% in decryption.

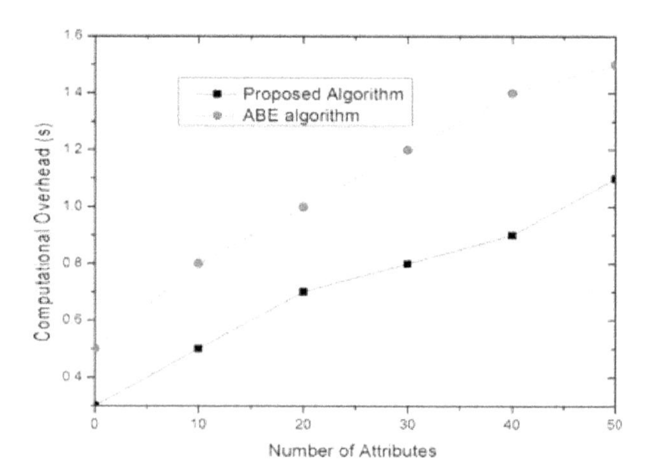

Fig. 4.2 Computational overhead in terms of Encryption

As a next step, the algorithms using the three operations such as creating a file, reading a file, and writing a file are evaluated. The performance is evaluated using the numberof waiting requests for a particular period. Three algorithms are considered for

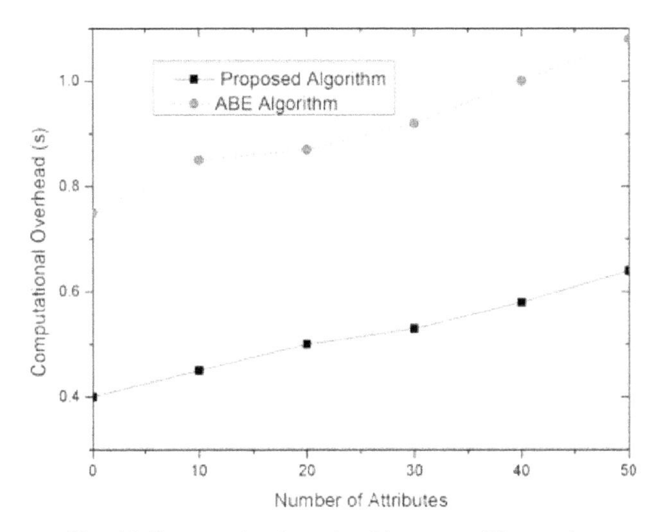

Fig. 4.3 Computational overhead in terms of Decryption

performance evaluation. The first one is the proposed algorithm which is a combination of AES and CP-ABE algorithms. These condone is Plutus (Kallahalla et al., 2003) which uses the same key for both encryption and decryption. The third one is SiRiUS (Goh et al., 2003) where each file in the model is associated with meta-data along with their access control mechanisms. In this algorithm, an encryption key is encrypted using the public key of the user. From Figure 4.4, it is observed that the computation over head of the proposed algorithm and Plutus is almost the same. But, the SiRiUS algorithm has more computation overhead. It is based on the number of creation operations generated by the authorized users. The heart rated at a is taken as a sample for simulation.

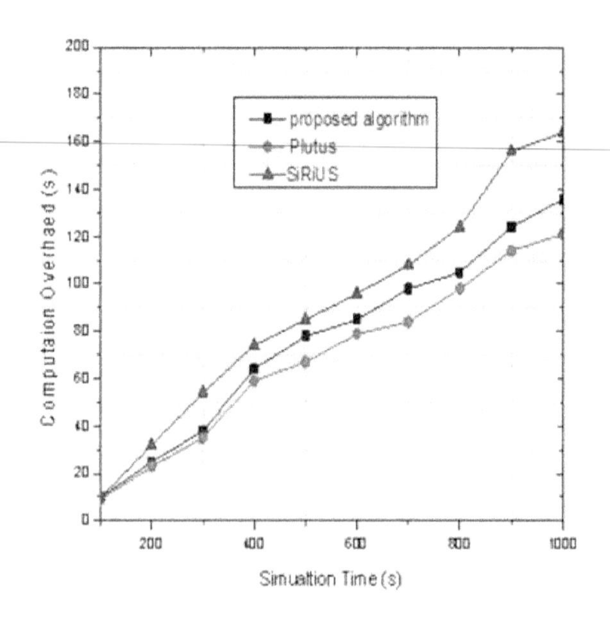

Fig. 4.4 Computational overhead interms of Create, Read, and Write Access Policies

In Figure 4.5, modifications are done to the access policies and the simulation iscarried out with three algorithms. In this case, it is observed that the proposed algorithm achieved higher performance compared to the Plutus (Kallahalla et al, 2003) and SiRiUS (Goh et al., 2003). In Plutus, the overhead is caused due to the change in the access policies which results in the re-encryption process of files. In SiRiUS, the re-encryption is carried for both files as well as for meta-data. The proposed algorithm avoids all these issues by managing the key expiration time and also the access policies are assigned temporarily to the users.

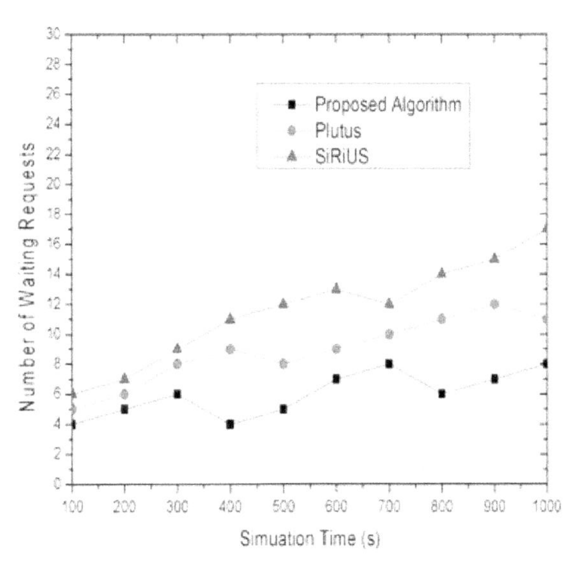

Fig. 4.5 Number of Waiting Requests Vs Simulation Time

The Encryption Time(ET) along with Decryption Times(DT) graphical illustration is exhibited in Figure 4.6.It examines the proposed and also the existing algorithm's ET. While the total sensor nodes are 200, 4.157 seconds are taken by the proposed method for converting the data (input) into ciphertext data, however, the prevailing research methods take 7.845 s for Plutus and 6.873s for SiRiUS. Only lesser time is taken by the proposed work for encrypting the data aimed at the remaining node count also. Figure 4.7 deems the proposed and the existing algorithm's DT. Here also, lesser time is taken by the proposed method for the decryption of data, for example, the proposed method takes 4.127 s for decrypting the data when the sensor node count is 200. The existent research methods require more time. The ET and also DT's overall analysis exhibits that lesser time is needed by the proposed method analogized to the existent research methodologies.

Table 4.4 Performance Analysis of secure data transfer based on encryption and Decryption time

Number of Nodes	Encryption Time (s)			Decryption Time (s)		
	Proposed Algorithm	Plutus	SiRiUS	Proposed Algorithm	Plutus	SiRiUS
40	2.814	3.908	4.825	2.813	3.97	4.82
80	2.975	5.985	5.012	2.864	5.65	5.42
120	3.145	7.025	5.754	3.138	6.99	5.96
160	3.765	7.412	6.128	3.784	7.54	6.12
200	4.157	7.845	6.873	4.127	8.10	6.97

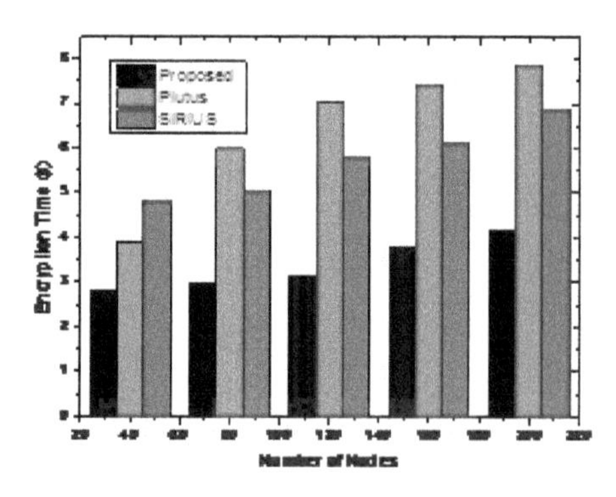

Fig. 4.6 Number of Nodes Vs Encryption Time

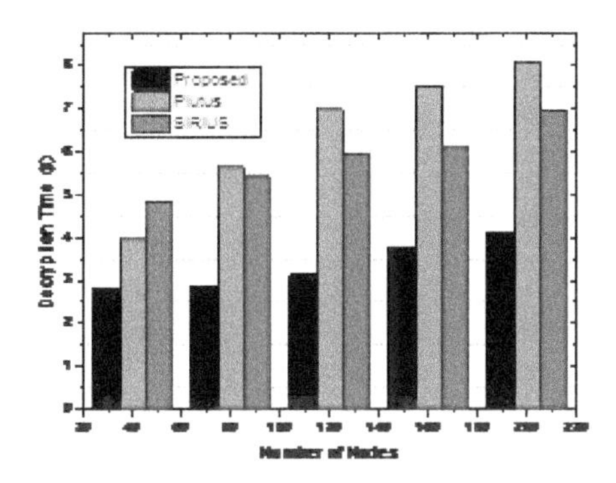

Fig. 4.7 Number of Nodes Vs Decryption Time

Figure 4.6 and Fig 4.7 shows Graphical representation of performance analysis of proposed algorithm-based secure data transfer with the existing algorithms in terms of encryption time and decryption time.
Table 4.5 examines the security level. Therein, the security level is poor for the prevailing Plutus algorithm, and a higher security level is attained by the proposed technique, analogized to the existing methods and is shown in Figure 4.8.

Table 4.5 Performance analysis of secure data transfer based on security level

Algorithm	Security Level
Proposed method	97.5%
Plutus	91.3 %
SiRiUS	94.6 %

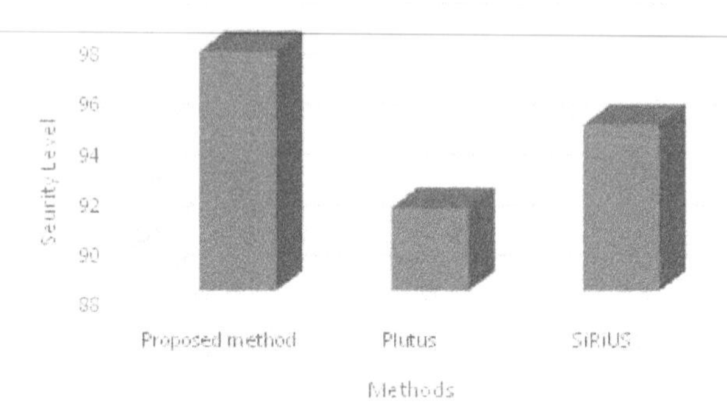

Fig. 4.8 Secure Data Transfer based on Security level

4.7 Summary

This chapter addressed the issue of data management in Medical-IoT. An efficient architecture that uses a cloud environment to store the data dynamically is developed. The next proposal is the security model that avoids the security issues of medical data and provides confidentiality, integrity with any user interventions. An efficient access control mechanism is developed by combining symmetric cryptography and attribute-based encryption. This hybrid algorithm reduced the computation over head at the time of the encryption and decryption process. The experimental analysis proved the efficiency of the proposed algorithm in terms of scalability, security, and access-control.

CHAPTER 5

ADAPTIVE AUTHENTICATION SCHEME BASED ON THE USER MOBILITY IN MEDICAL-IoT

5.1 Introduction

The industry of networking has been experiencing IoT for the past few years since its emergence as a technology of prime significance. It serves as the connecting network for clients, vehicles, home devices, etc, via tags, sensors and actuators. IoT-enabled communications among these areas utilize the digital form. The home automation, health care, vehicle systems and similar structures in the global scenario function with more capability and the support offered by IoT(Escobaret al.,2017). In many of the M-IoT applications, generally the doctors as well as the patients are in fixed locations where the services may be offered, but at times they are in a mobile situation. The prime drive behind this task is providing security as well as privacy to the doctors as well as patients when they move around or travel.

Medical-IoT(M-IoT) is making phenomenal advancements in communication between doctors as well as patients. Such an entity is utilized in home-based treatment for patients in improving their quality of life. However, security and privacy in the M-IoT are the major issues that still needs to be considered. They are prone to be disclosed by the insecure network available with the health care professionals or at the service place (Yin et al., 2016). The communicating services under the wireless type of medical services are steeply increasing in use for promoting health care services as well as in applications. Various problems of security needs associated with the M-IoT need solutions. Health care and medical data must be secured utilizing the mechanisms of cryptography as well as the principles of authentication.Several research scholars have made proposals of different mechanisms for addressing the authentication in M-IoT (Li et al., 2014). Yet, there is still scope to improvethe security in M-IoT.

The stated security challenges will increase when the clients locations are changed by them. The prime drive behind this task is providing security as well asprivacy to the doctors as well as patients when they move around or travel. The target of this proposed framework is to authenticate the clients while they are moving or traveling and to compute the performance metrics.

- To propose authentication and authorization mechanism for medical IoT based on the user mobility.

- To compute various performance metrics like computation time, communication overhead of the devised protocol and compare against other existing protocols.

Proposed different authentication mechanisms between the patient and doctor who are available in different regions. The proposed mechanism provides the authentication, anonymity, data integrity and mutual authentication. It also uses symmetric encryption techniques to preserve the security in Medical-IoT. The performance of the authentication mechanism is tested with real time environment.
The remaining portions of the chapter are structured in the following manner: Section5.2 narrates the recent works related to the medical IoT. Section 5.3 describes the proposed framework for authenticating the clients while they are moving or traveling. Section 5.4 explains the analysis of security in the proposed model. Section 5.5 deals with the experimental analysis of the authentication mechanisms. Section 5.6 contains the conclusions of the research work.

5.2 Security Requirements and Proposed Framework

In this section, the security requirements and proposed framework are discussed along with the communication mechanism between the participants.

5.2.1 Network Model

As a generalized situation, the health care authority, doctors as well as the patients in the medical system are considered here. The maintaining of the server for authentication is in the Medical-IoT where the authority for health care is present. The registration of clients is done under this server kept for authentication. The stated model in the proposal takes care of preserving the privacy as well as the security even during the clients mobility. Figure5.1 depicts the model in the proposal. It has remote as well as local servers offering the needed services based on the status of the clients. In the

Table 5.1 Nomenclature

Symbol	Description
L	Local Server
R	Remote Server
H_A	Healthcare Authority
P	Patient
D	Doctor
X_i	X might be the patient or doctor and i the user ID
$X_{i.ID.j}$	j denotes the subliminal ID of the user I
$K_{X.Y}$	Secret key shared between x and y
Z_R	Remote Server
(..)k	Data encryption using the symmetric key encryption mechanism
N_X	Nonce generated by X
TS	Time stamp
T_{key}	Temporary key
TKT	Ticket
Tkn	Token

model shown, the clients are free to move around any location and can securely do the necessary communications.

5.2.2 Preliminaries

The model maintains three prime servers namely the local server, remote server and user registration via the authority for health care:

Local server (L): L servers location is in the network of the home area. It has the responsibility for storing the doctor's and patient's IDs and symmetric secret key $K_{X.L}$. This key is shared between user X and local server L. The routing table Z_L is maintained by L which contains the users real IDs and corresponding subliminal IDs and provides a mapping of them. It also maintains the secret key $K_{L,R}$ to create the communication between the local server L and remote server R.

Remote server (R): The location of R is outside the home area network and stores a secret key $K_{L,R}$ .This key is shared between L and R. It also stores the secret key$K_{RU,R}$ that is being shared between the remote user R_U and R and maintains the routing table Z_R.

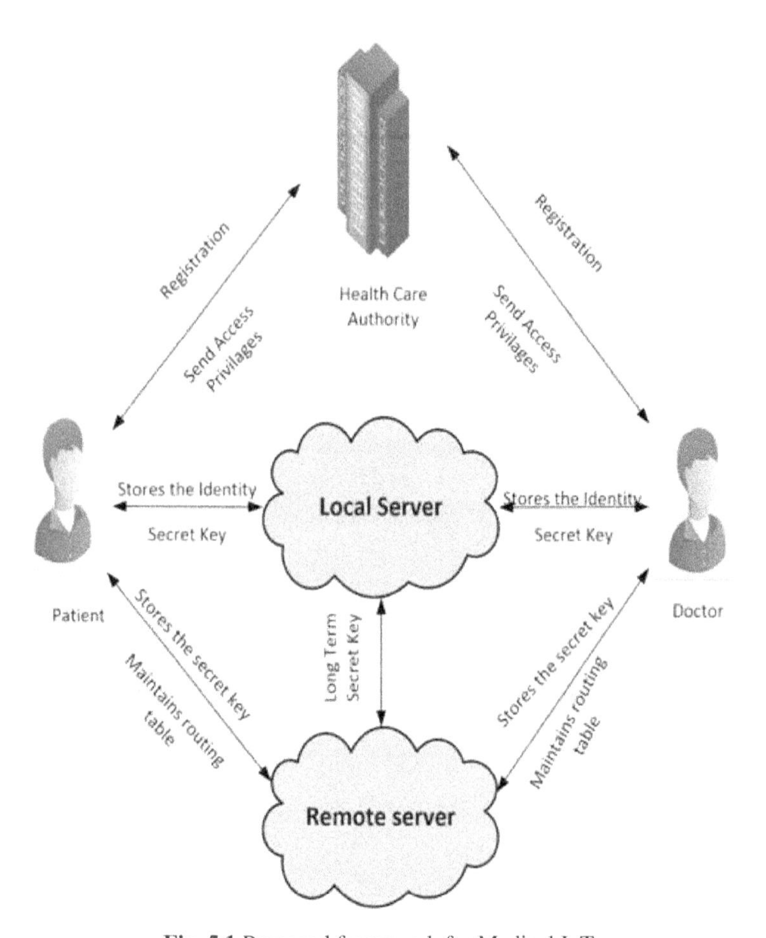

Fig. 5.1 Proposed framework for Medical IoT

Health Care Authority (H_A): H_A deals with both the doctor as well as the patient registrations. The patient performs only one-time registration with L. The main reason for the patient registration is to register the ID along with the setup of secret key $K_{P,L}$. This is obtainable by their own password. The patient's ID is stored in the table as well as mapped with the subliminal ID. The latter will be the phone number or IP address, depending on the type of system. The doctors registration is very similar to that of the patients registration, except the subliminal IDs are not used for them. The doctors ID is registered under L and gets the secret key $K_{d,L}$.

5.2.3 The Proposed Authentication Protocols

In this research work, three conditions are considered to establish a secure communication channel between doctors and patients either in a different location or in the same place. These conditions are being analyzed in the proposed authentication protocol in both wired and wireless communication.
a) P-L-D Condition

b) P-R-L-D Condition

c) P-R-DCondition

a) P-L-Dcondition

In this condition, Patient P, as well as doctor D,communicate with each other through the local server L placed in the same location i.e., local server L which is managed by the health care authority H_A. There are a couple of phases in such a situation, ticket generation and consultation phase. Figure 5.2 shows the ticket generation and consultation phase in the P-L-D condition.
1. Ticket Generation Phase
The prime objective of this module is to provide communication and permit mutual authentication between the users. Such secure communication is carried out through the trusted local server L by patient P as well as doctor D.The implementation of sub sequent steps are done by P and L to obtain a consultation from D. P can communicate with D utilizing the ticket $TKT_{P,D}$.

This can be carried out by the following step:

$$TKT = [K_s, P, P_{i,ID.1}, D, TS]K_{d.L} \tag{5.1}$$

2. Consultation Phase

In this consulting phase, patient P sends the TKT to doctor D for ensuring the consultancy. D confirms the consent to the request by sending the reply to patient P. The communication between P and D is carried via the trusted server L. The messages exchanged between P and D are encrypted by utilizing the secret key Ks. The procedure for the proposed authentication protocol in the P-L-D conditionis as given below.

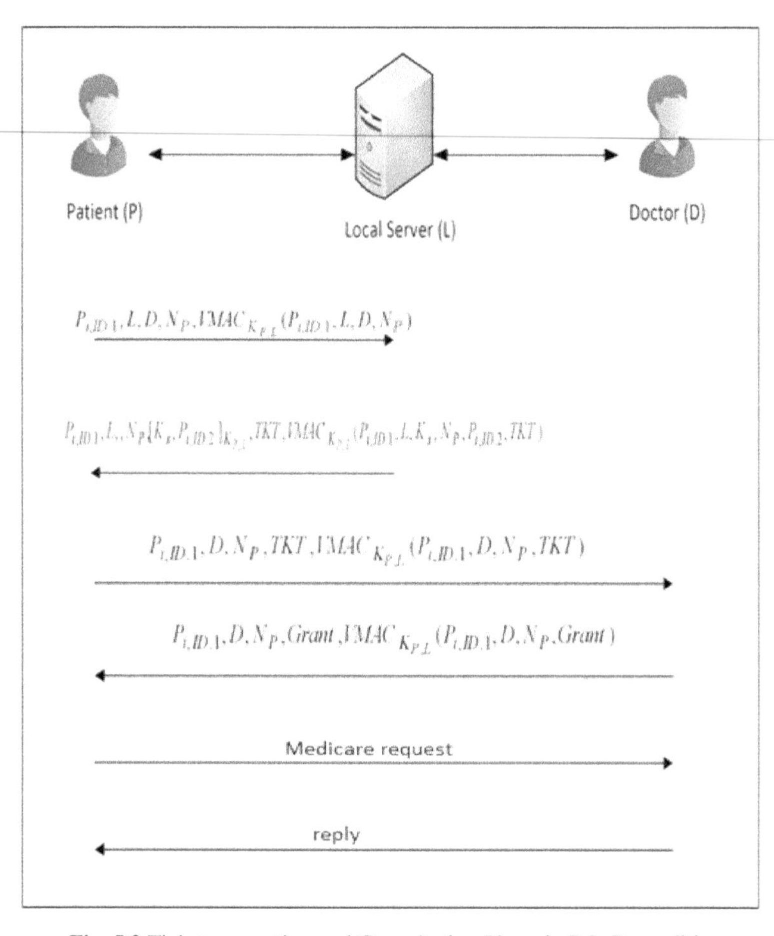

Fig. 5.2 Ticket generation and Consultation Phase in P-L-D condition

i. $P \rightarrow L: P_{i,ID.1}, L, D, N_P, VMAC_{K_{P,L}}(P_{i,ID.1}, L, D, N_P)$

ii. $L \rightarrow P: P_{i,ID.1}, L., N_P, [K_s, P_{i,ID.2}]_{K_{P,L}}, TKT,$

$VMAC_{K_{P,L}}(P_{i,ID.1}, L, K_s, N_P, P_{i,ID.2}, TKT)$

iii. $P \rightarrow L \rightarrow D : P_{i,ID.1}, D, N_P, TKT, VMAC_{K_{P,L}}(P_{i,ID.1}, D, N_P, TKT)$

iv. $D \rightarrow L \rightarrow P : P_{i,ID.1}, D, N_P, Grant, VMAC_{K_{P,L}}(P_{i,ID.1}, D, N_P, Grant)$

v. $P \rightarrow L \rightarrow D:$ $Medicarequest$

vi. $D \rightarrow L \rightarrow P: Reply$

b)P-R-L-D Condition

In this condition, patient P is positioned in a remote location while doctor D is in the home location which is shown in Figure 5.3. Now patient P sends a request to consult doctor D. In this situation, patient P must contact the local server L to get the secret key K. But this is not possible without support from the remote server R.

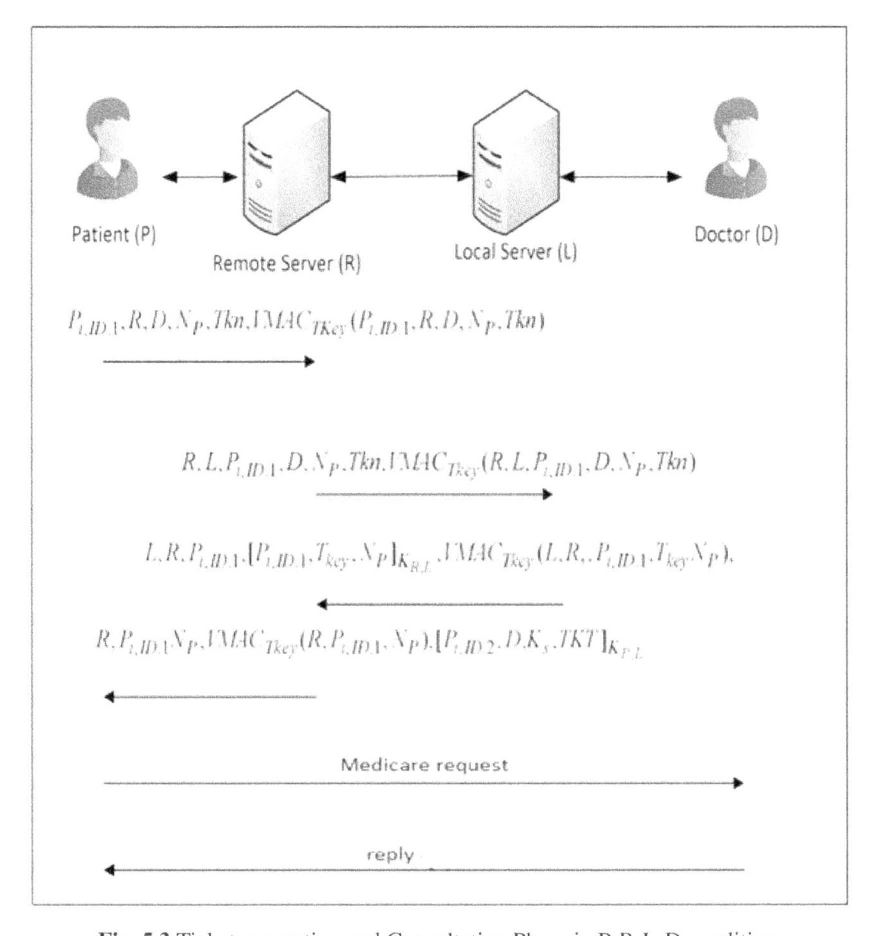

Fig. 5.3 Ticket generation and Consultation Phase in P-R-L-D condition

Therefore, the servers of local L and remote R must share the long-term secret key K. Now, authentication is carried out through the remote server R towards local server Land patient P and finally onwards to D.

1. Ticket Generation Phase

The module explains that P is in a remotely located place. Prequires assistance through R, a remote server for consulting D, the doctor. Now authenticating is done between P and D with the aid of local server L as well as remote server R. The prime question here is the way R is validates theauthentication of P where R has no information regarding P. R will obtain the temporary secret key by applying the data encrypting on what was received from P. L shares the key with R for validating the authentication of P.

2. Consultation Phase

Now, patient P contacts doctor D with the available ticket. The communicating way between the P and R is similar to the P-L-D condition, but the variation is Rand L are associated in the communicating method.

c) P-R-D Condition

i. $P \rightarrow R\colon P_{i.ID.1}, R, D, N_P, Tkn, VMAC_{TKey}(P_{i.ID.1}, R, D, N_P, Tkn)$

$$Where\ Tkn = [P_{i.ID.1}, L, R, N_P]_{K_{P.L}}$$

ii. $R \rightarrow L\colon R, L, P_{i.ID.1}, D, N_P, Tkn, VMAC_{Tkey}(R, L, P_{i.ID.1}, D, N_P, Tkn)$

iii. $L \rightarrow R : L, R, P_{i.ID.1}, [P_{i.ID.1}, T_{key}, N_P]_{K_{R.L}}, VMAC_{Tkey}(L, R., P_{i.ID.1}, T_{key}, N_P),$

$$[P_{i.ID.2}, D.K_s, TKT]_{K_{P.L}}\ where\ TKT = [P, P_{i.ID.1}, D, K_s, T]_{K_{d.L}}$$

iv. $R \rightarrow P : R, P_{i.ID.1} N_P, VMAC_{Tkey}(R, P_{i.ID.1}, N_P).[P_{i.ID.2}, D.K_s, TKT]_{K_{P.L}}$

In this condition patient P as well as the doctor D are in the remote place. The ticket generating phase for patient P is similar to the P-R-L-D situation. The local server L authenticates the doctor D with the aid of the remote server R.

The patient P as well as doctor D require to contact the local server L for secured communication. This is due to the fact that the remote server R does not have any stored information for verifying the credentials of P as well as D. The patient authenticating way is the same as the second condition. So, R authenticates D for establishing secure communication with P. Here R verifies D by obtaining the support of L. The procedure to authenticate and then to consult a doctor D is shown in figure 5.4:

Authentication Phase: To start with, the doctor D contacts the remote server R with token Tkn and temporary key T key which are received from local server L. Next, the remote server R forwards token Tkn to the local server L for verifying the information regarding doctor D and requests temporary key Tkey associated with doctor D. Subsequently, the local server L forwards Tkey to remote server R for validating the doctors authenticity D by the remote server R. Finally, R does the verification of the doctors authenticity D.

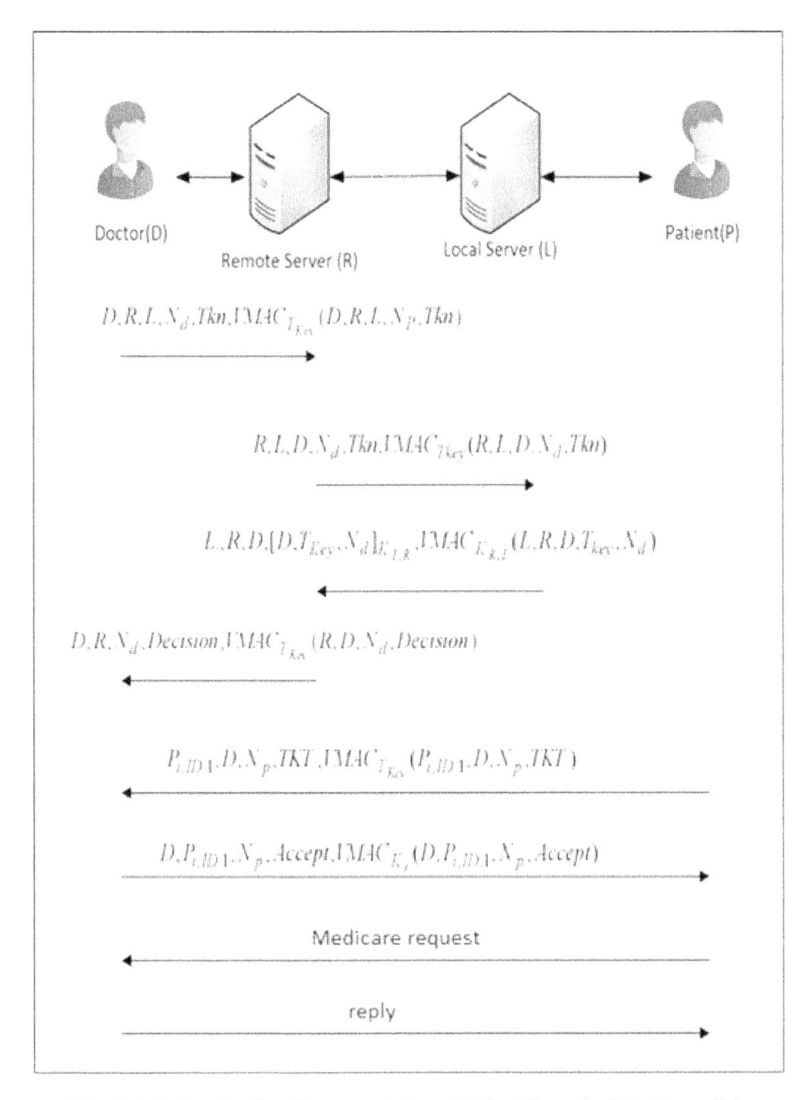

Fig. 5.4 Authentication Phase and Consultation Phase in P-R-D condition

i. $D \rightarrow R: D, R, L, N_d, Tkn, VMAC_{T_{Key}}(D, R, L, N_P, Tkn)$

$$where Tkn = [D, R, L, N_P]_{K_{d,L}} \quad and \ T_{key} = f(K_{d,L}, N_d, D)$$

ii. $R \rightarrow L: R, L, D, N_d, Tkn, VMAC_{T_{key}}(R, L, D, N_d, Tkn)$

iii. $L \rightarrow R: L., R, D, [D, T_{Key}, N_d]_{K_{L,R}}, VMAC_{K_{R,L}}(L, R, D, T_{key}, N_d)$

iv. $R \rightarrow D: D, R, N_d, Decision, VMAC_{T_{Key}}(R, D, N_d, Decision)$

v. $P \rightarrow R \rightarrow D: P_{i,ID.1}, D, N_p, TKT, VMAC_{T_{Key}}(P_{i,ID.1}, D, N_p, TKT)$

vi. $D \rightarrow R \rightarrow P: D, P_{i,ID.1}, N_p, Accept, VMAC_{K_i}(D, P_{i,ID.1}, N_p, Accept)$

vii. $P \rightarrow R \rightarrow D: Medicare \quad request$

viii. $D \rightarrow R \rightarrow P: reply$

5.3 SecurityAnalysis

Under the aforementioned security assumptions, the proposed protocols possess the following security properties defined earlier which considered only the outside adversaries including outsiders who are not registered with the system and insiders who have been registered with their local server but are involved in the protocol execution. All adversaries can launch active attacks. For simplicity, the adversary is denoted by A.

5.3.1 Replay Attacks

The mechanism of authenticating in the proposal utilizes the nonce when the two parties communicate. On each occasion, a fresh random number is generated utilizing then once. It ensures data freshness after completing the session. The data from the prior session is not utilized in the present session, as the former sessions n once differs from the present session. This ensures that the data is new.

5.3.2 Anonymity

The user anonymity is achieved with the subliminal ID of the user. In the proposedmethod, even if a user, say A, has his own key, he cannot know the other users' identities, though he can obtain the identity of his communication partner. The reason is threefold: (1) A subliminal identity is used only for one round of the protocol and a new subliminal ID is transmitted to the user securely. (2) The new subliminal ID is encrypted by the local server, therefore, only the corresponding user can decrypt it. (3) The proposed method also offers patient untraceability, which means that a patient cannot be traced back with the previous communication transcripts. The reason is that the subliminal ID updated when a communication session completed.

5.3.3 Data Integrity

Preserving the integrity of the data in the proposed model is carried out by utilizing the algorithm of virtual message authentication code (VMAC). This algorithm is a mechanism of authentication which utilizes the hash function for secure communication. The VMAC generates the long-term secret key. This can be shared between the client and the local server. The clients who have the key can calculate the value of VMAC and establish communication. The stated procedure preserves the integrity of data in the model.

5.3.4 Data Confidentiality

Patients who live in remote areas can communicate with the healthcare provider and benefit from doctor consultations. Data are confidential matter and preserving it is possible. Here, the sharing of the long-term secret key by the client is sent to the local server. For data retrieval, the client submits the key to the local server. The decryption of the data are done with the key. Thus maintaining data confidentiality is realized in the proposed method.

5.4 Performance Analysis

The proposed model is implemented in Boto3 which is an AWS SDK used by python 3.3. The AWS EC2 instances use the Xeon CPU @ 3.3GHz with 16GB RAM and Linux 16.04 OS. The sample code to deploy the instances in Boto3 is given as follows:

```
for i in ec2.instances.all():
ifi.state['Name'] == 'stopped':
i.start()
```

The performance of the proposed authentication model is evaluated using the security features which are given in Table 5.1. The algorithms help to compare the performance of the proposed model with the existing mechanisms (Chiouet al., 2016; Chen etal., 2014; Chenget al.,2017).

Table 5.2 Comparison of Security Parameters

Security Parameter	**Chiou etal., (2016)**	**Chen etal., (2014)**	**Cheng etal., (2017)**	**Proposed Method**
Restricting replay attacks	YES	YES	YES	YES
Protecting the user privacy	YES	NO	NO	YES
Mutual authentication	NO	NO	NO	YES
Data confidentiality	YES	YES	NO	YES
Data Integrity	YES	NO	NO	YES

In Chiou etal.,(2017), the authors failed to achieve mutual authentication in the cloud telemedicine system. In Chen et al., (2014), the model failed to achieve user privacy, mutual authentication, and data integrity. Furthermore, Cheng et al., (2017) failed to satisfy user privacy, authentication, confidentiality and integrity.

Table 5.3 Computational cost details of server

Number of Doctors	**Computational load on server(ns)**			
	Proposed Algorithm	**cheng et al**	**chen et al**	**chiou et al**
5	500	920	920	1000
10	1200	1850	1850	2200
15	1556	2680	2680	2954
20	2358	3547	3547	3857
25	2480	4250	4250	4855
30	2985	4847	4847	5540
35	3240	5652	5652	6874
40	3955	6845	6845	7580

Figure 5.5 shows the computation cost of the server incurred at the time of performing the authentication of patients and doctors simultaneously. It is observed that the time taken by the proposed method for authentication of users is less compared to the other existing mechanisms. Figure 5.6 shows the computation cost of a complete one-round procedure from the patient authentication phase to the doctor reply phase. It

is proved that the proposed method is efficient for providing mutual authentication in P-L-D, P-L-R-D and P-R-D conditions.

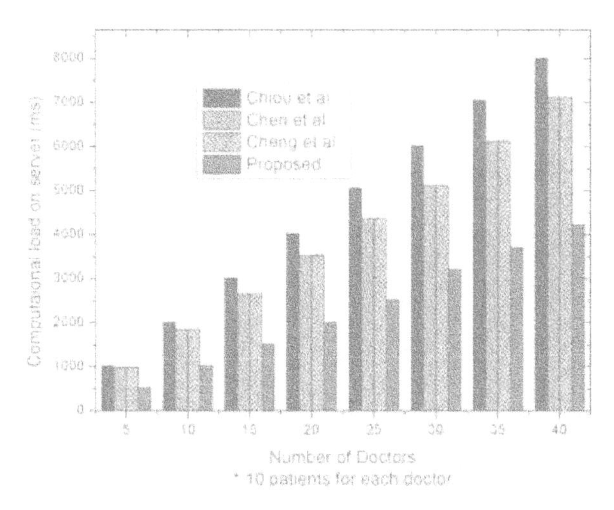

Fig. 5.5 Comparison of Computational Cost in Server

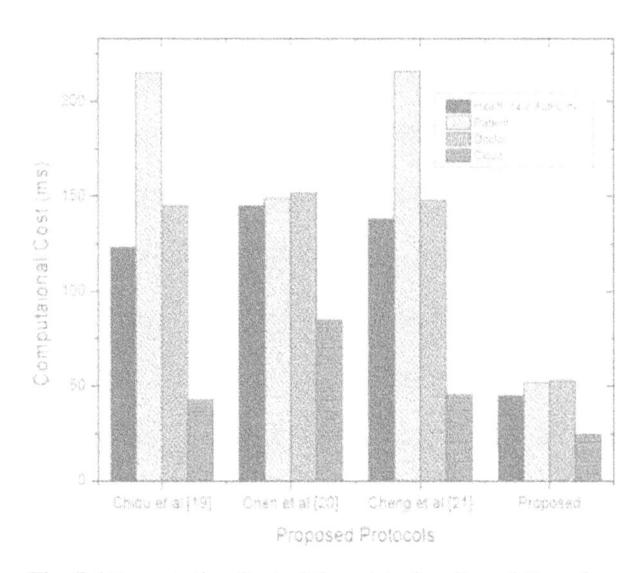

Fig. 5.6 Computation Cost of Complete One Round Procedure

5.5 Summary

This chapter contains the mechanism of authentication in the proposal for the Medical-IoT. It provides a secure channel of communication from doctor to patient in local or remote locations. Communicating in the wireless and wired types of devices is possible among users. The mechanism of authentication in the proposal realized confidentiality, anonymity, integrity as well as mutual authentication. Added to it clients mobility is also handled. That aspect is not offered in other similar existing methods. The proposed model is economically viable as it is cost-effective, for example, in the cost of computation. It has high speed and it utilizes the symmetric key encryption mechanism.

CHAPTER 6

CONCLUSION AND FUTURE WORK

6.1 Conclusion

Security is commonly described as the interplay of confidentiality, integrity, and availability, potentially extended with additional constructs such as accountability, auditability, trustworthiness, or non-repudiation. Privacy issues may lead to different kinds of negative effects for individuals. Also from a legal point of view it is important to ensure privacy of personal data. Combining and processing seemingly innocent data may introduce privacy problems for IoT-users. Especially in the IoT, privacy problems may arise. Privacy can be grouped into several "objectives". The application of wireless devices has led to a significant improvement in the quality and delivery of care in telemedicine systems. Patients who live in remote areascan communicate with the healthcare provider and benefit from doctor consultations.

However, it has been a challenge to provide a secure telemedicine system, which captures users and patients privacy. To overcome these issues, as a first contribution, the proposed model considers three modules, namely, two-way authentication, symmetric key generation and disjoint multipath data transmission. Enhanced symmetric key encryption mechanism is developedby managing the three-way handshake between the gateways and the cloud servers. The dis joint multipath data transmission provides high security by fragmenting the encrypted data. The experiment analysis validated that the algorithm in the proposal is capable of authentication and also decreases the delay for data transmission.

In the second contribution, this thesis addressed the issue of data management in Medical-IoT by developing an efficient architecture that uses a cloud environment to store the data dynamically. Next, a security model that avoids the security issues of medical data and provides confidentiality, integrity with any user interventions is proposed. An efficient access control mechanism is developed by combining symmetric cryptography and attribute based encryption. This hybrid algorithm reduced the computation over head at the time of the encryption and decryption process. The experimental analysis validated the capability of the algorithm in the proposal as far as security, scalability and access control are concerned.

In the final contribution, a proposal is made for an authentication mechanism to the Medical-IoT. It provides a secure communication channel from doctor to patient in a local place or remote position. The communication may be through wireless or wired type of devices among the customers. The mechanism of authentication in the proposal realized confidentiality, anonymity, integrity as well as mutual authentication. Apart from this, there is a capability of handling the mobilityof clients. This is not offered in the existing mechanisms in use. The mechanism in the proposal has minimal computation cost as well as high speed. It utilizes the symmetric key encryption mechanism.

6.2 Future Work

M-IoT has been given and received much attention of late. However, related standards and technical specifications are still evolving. Special application requirements of healthcare and more successful associated explorations are needed. Focus and concentration on accessing policies to the users and designing a mechanism for key distribution and recovery process will be the target of the upcoming research efforts. Future research may focus for example on how to determine what the main security and privacy objectives are in a specific situation, how to implement the guidelines, and how to evaluate their effectiveness. What would be interesting is a system with decentralized PEP and PDP, which is dynamically updatable, monitorable and transparent to users of devices, and allows software updates, but at the same time privacy preserving. What such a system would look like is hard to say. Advances have been made with SDN / NFV-based authentication and authorization. Very little is known however about these IoT technologys impact on privacy of users.
Beyond the growing market for healthcare IoT, the COVID-19 pandemic has spurred conversations around the future of IoT in healthcare and how it can safely connect healthcare professionals and patients. Hospitals and clinics were forced to quickly evaluate telehealth to continue to treat some patients without increasing their risk of infection by bringing them into care facilities. Hospitals are also under constant pressure to identify ways to reduce costs. Wearable devices that enable some patients to be treated and monitored at home could reduce the number of resources needed at the healthcare facility.

For blockchain-based solutions, access control polices are saved in a distributed ledger, privacy issues may arise as everybody may have an overview of a users or devices rights which have distributed, alternative methods for authentication that separate authentication from a natural users personal identity such as group signatures, attribute-based authentication, or alternative authentication measures (non-identity) such as multi-factor authentication may make identity attributes less visible to transmitting parties. Future research may focus on these areas, to find a balance between auditability, visibility, and transparency on the one hand and users privacy and unlinkability on the other.

REFERENCES

A.K. (2018), A hybrid model of internet of things and cloud computing to manage big data in health services application, Future generation computer systems, 86(3), 1383-1394.

Abbas, A. and Khan, S.U. (2014), A review on the state-of-the-art privacy-preserving approaches in the e-health clouds, IEEE Journal of Biomedical and Health Informatics, 18(4), 1431-1441.

Abdmeziem, M.R. and Tandjaoui, D. (2014), A cooperative end to end key management scheme for e-health applications in the context of internet of things. in Proceedings of the International Conference on Ad-Hoc Networks and Wireless, pp. 35-46.

Agu, E., Pedersen, P., Strong, D., Tulu, B., He, Q., Wang, L. and Li, Y. (2013), The smartphone as a medical device: Assessing enablers, benefits and challenges, in IEEE International Workshop of Internet-of-Things Networking and Control (IoT-NC) , pp. 48-52.

Ahmed, N., Kanhere, S.S. and Jha, S. (2005), The holes problem in wireless sensor networks: a survey, ACM SIGMOBILE Mobile Computing and Communications Review, 9(2), 4-18.

Airehrour, D., Gutierrez, J. and Ray, S.K. (2016), A lightweight trust design for IoT routing, in IEEE 14th International Conference on Dependable, Autonomic and Secure Computing,, pp. 552-557.

Airehrour, D., Gutierrez, J. and Ray, S.K. (2016), Securing RPL routing protocol from black hole attacks using a trust-based mechanism, in Proceedings of 26thInternational Telecommunication Networks and Applications Conference (ITNAC), pp. 115-120.

Alaba, F.A., Othman, M., Hashem, I.A.T. and Alotaibi, F. (2017), Internet of Things security: A survey, Journal of Network and Computer Applications, 88(1), 10-28.

Alpr, G., Batina, L., Batten, L., Moonsamy, V., Krasnova, A., Guellier, A. and Natgunanathan, I. (2016), New directions in IoT privacy using Attribute-based Authentication in Proceedings of the ACM International Conference on Computing Frontiers, pp. 461-466.

Alphand, O., Amoretti, M., Claeys, T., Dall'Asta, S., Duda, A., Ferrari, G., R'ousseau, F., Tourancheau, B., Veltri, L.and Zanichelli, F.(2018), IoT Chain: A Blockchain security architecture for the Internet of Things, in 2018 IEEE Wireless Communications and Networking Conference (WCNC), pp. 1-6.

Alur, R., Berger, E., Drobnis, A.W., Fix, L., Fu, K., Hager, G.D., Lopresti, D., Nahrstedt, K., Mynatt, E., Patel, S. and Rexford, J. (2016), Systems computing challenges in the Internet of Things, arXiv preprint arXiv:1604.02980.

Anirudh, M., Thileeban, S.A. and Nallathambi, D.J. (2017), Use of honeypots for mitigating DoS attacks targeted on IoT networks, in International Conference on Computer, Communication and Signal processing (ICCCSP), pp. 1-4.

Attribute-based multi-keyword search over encrypted personal health records in multi-owner setting, Journal of Medical Systems, 40(11), pp. 246-246.

Atzori, L., Iera, A. and Morabito, G. (2010), The internet of things: A survey, Computer Networks, 54(15), 2787-2805. Atzori, L., Iera, A. and Morabito, G. (2016), The Internet of things: A survey, Computer Networks, 54(15), 2787-2805.

B. and Andreescu, S. (2015), Health monitoring and management using Internet-of-Things (IoT) sensing with cloud-based processing: Opportunities and challenges, in IEEE International Conference on Services Computing, pp. 285-292.

B.W. John Bethencourt, Amit Sahai, Cp-abe library,URL: Online at http://acsc.cs.utexas.edu /cpabe/.

Bacis, E., De Capitani di Vimercati, S., Foresti, S., Paraboschi, S., Rosa, M. and Samarati, P. (2016), MixandSlice: Efficient access revocation in the cloud., in Proceedings of the 2016 ACM SIGSAC Conference on Computer and Communications Security, pp. 217-228.

Bae, G.C. and Shin, K.W. (2016), An efficient hardware implementation of lightweight block cipher algorithm CLEFIA for IoT security applications, Journal of the Korea Institute of Information and Communication Engineering, 20(2), 351-358.

Baker, S.B., Xiang, W. and Atkinson, I. (2017), Internet of things for Smart Healthcare: Technologies, Challenges, and Opportunities, IEEE Access, 5(4), 26521- 26544.

Bamasag, O.O. and Youcef-Toumi, K. (2015), Towards continuous authentication in Internet of Things based on secret sharing scheme, in Proceedings of the WESS'15: Workshop on Embedded Systems Security, pp. 1-8.

Bassi, A., Bauer, M., Fiedler, M., van Kranenburg, R., Lange, S., Meissner, S. and Kramp, T. (2013), Enabling things to talk 379 Springer Nature, 10(1), 90-94.

Bazzani, M., Conzon, D., Scalera, A., Spirito, M.A. and Trainito, C.I. (2012), Enabling the IoT paradigm in e-health solutions through the VIRTUS middleware. in IEEE 11th international conference on trust, security and privacy in computing and communications , IEEE, pp. 1954-1959.

Bennett, J., Rokas, O. and Chen, L. (2017), Healthcare in the smart home: A study of Past, Present and Future, Sustainability, 9(5), p.840.

Bernabe, J.B., Ramos, J.L.H. and Gomez, A.F.S. (2016), TACIoT: Multidimensional trust-aware access control system for the Internet of Things, Soft Computing, 20(5), pp.1763-1779.

Bethencourt, J., Sahai, A. and Waters, B. (2007), Ciphertext-policy attribute-based encryption, in 2007 IEEE symposium on security and privacy (SP'07), IEEE, pp. 321-334.

Bethencourt, J., Sahai, A. and Waters, B. (2007), Ciphertext-policy attribute-based encryption, in 2007 IEEE symposium on security and privacy (SP'07), pp. 321-334.

Bezawada, B., Liu, A.X., Jayaraman, B., Wang, A.L. and Li, R. (2015), Privacy-preserving string matching for cloud computing, in IEEE 35th International Conference on Distributed Computing Systems, pp. 609-618.

Bio Assist. Available online: https://bioassist.gr/ (accessed on 22 June 2019). Boxwala, A.A., Kim, J., Grillo, J.M. and Ohno-Machado, L. (2011), Using statistical and machine learning to help institutions detect suspicious access to electronic health records, Journal of the American Medical Informatics Association, 18(4), 498-505.

Bresson, E., Chevassut, O. and Pointcheval, D. (2002), Dynamic group Diffie- Hellman key exchange under standard assumptions, in International conference on the theory and applications of cryptographic techniques Springer, Berlin, Heidelberg, pp. 321-336.

Bui, N., Bressan, N. and Zorzi, M. (2012), Interconnection of body area networks to a communications infrastructure: An architectural study, in European Wireless 2012; 18th European Wireless Conference, pp. 1-8.

Cao, N., Wang, C., Li, M., Ren, K. and Lou, W. (2013), Privacy-preserving multi-keyword ranked search over encrypted cloud data, IEEE Transactions on parallel and distributed systems, 25(1), 222-233.

Castillejo, P., Martinez, J.F., Rodriguez-Molina, J. and Cuerva, A. (2013), Integration of wearable devices in a wireless sensor network for an E-health application, IEEE Wireless Communications, 20(4), 38-49.

Cekerevac, Z., Dvorak, Z., Prigoda, L. and Cekerevac, P. (2017), Man in the Middle Attacks and the Internet of ThingsSecurity and economic risk. FBIM Trans, 5(1), 25-35.

Chae, C.J., Choi, K.N., Choi, K., Yae, Y.H. and Shin, Y. (2015), The Extended Authentication Protocol using E-mail Authentication in OAuth 2.0 Protocol for Secure Granting of User Access, Journal of Internet Computing and Services, 16(1), 21-28.

Chen, C.L., Yang, T.T. and Shih, T.F. (2014), A secure medical data exchange protocol based on cloud environment, Journal of Medical Systems, 38(9), 112-114.

Chen, C.L., Yang, T.T., Chiang, M.L. and Shih, T.F. (2014), A privacy authentication scheme based on cloud for medical environment, Journal of Medical Systems, 38(11), 143-144.

Chen, M., Qian, Y., Mao, S., Tang, W. and Yang, X. (2016), Software-defined mobile networks security, Mobile Networks and Applications, 21(5), 729-743.

Chen, M., Zhang, Y., Li, Y., Hassan, M.M. and Alamri, A. (2015), AIWAC: Affective interaction through wearable computing and cloud technology, IEEE Wireless Communications, 22(1), pp.20-27.

Chen, Y., Nyemba, S. and Malin, B. (2012), Auditing medical records accesses via healthcare interaction networks, in AMIA Annual Symposium Proceedings American Medical Informatics Association. , p. 93.

Cheng, Q., Zhang, X. and Ma, J. (2017), ICASME: An improved cloud-based authentication scheme for medical environment, Journal of Medical Systems, 41(3), pp.1-14.

Chiou, S.Y., Ying, Z. and Liu, J. (2016), Improvement of a privacy Authentication scheme based on cloud for Medical environment, Journal of Medical Systems, 40(4), 101-101.

Chiuchisan, I., Chiuchisan, I. and Dimian, M. (2015), Internet of Things for e-Health: An approach to medical applications, in International Workshop on Computational Intelligence for Multimedia Understanding (IWCIM), pp. 1-5.

Chiuchisan, I., Chiuchisan, I. and Dimian, M. (2015), Internet of Things for e-Health: An approach to medical applications, in International Workshop on Computational Intelligence for Multimedia Understanding (IWCIM), pp. 1-5.

Dai, Y., Wang, H., Zhou, Z. and Jin, Z. (2016), Research on medical image encryption in telemedicine systems, Technology and Health Care, 24(s2), S435-S442.

Dohr, A., Modre-Opsrian, R., Drobics, M., Hayn, D. and Schreier, G. (2010), The Internet of Things for ambient assisted living, in IEEE seventh international conference on information technology: new generations , pp. 804-809.

Du, W., Deng, J., Han, Y.S., Varshney, P.K., Katz, J. and Khalili, A. (2005), A Pairwise Key Pre Distribution Scheme for Wireless Sensor Networks, ACM Transactions on Information and System Security (TISSEC), 8(2), 228-258.

Du, W., Deng, J., Han, Y.S., Varshney, P.K., Katz, J. and Khalili, A. (2005), A pairwise key pre-distribution scheme for wireless sensor Networks., ACM Transactions on Information and System Security (TISSEC), 8(2), 228-258.

Elhoseny, M., Abdelaziz, A., Salama, A.S., Riad, A.M., Muhammad, K. and Sangaiah, Ericsson, T.L. and Johansson, H., 1935. Telefonaktiebolaget LM Ericsson. URL: https://www.ericsson.com/en/mobility-report/internet-of-thingsforecast.

Forsstrm, S., Kanter, T. and sterberg, P. (2012), Ubiquitous secure interactions with intelligent artifacts on the Internet of Things, in Proceedings of IEEE 11th International Conference on Trust, Security and Privacy in Computing and Communications, pp. 1520-1524.

Forsstrm, S., Kanter, T. and sterberg, P. (2012), Ubiquitous secure interactions with intelligent artifacts on the Internet of Things, in IEEE 11th International Conferenceon Trust, Security and Privacy in Computing and Communications, pp. 1520-1524.

Forsstrm, S., Kanter, T.and sterberg, P. (2012), Ubiquitous secure interactions with intelligent artifacts on the Internet-of-Things in IEEE 11th International Conference on Trust, Security and Privacy in Computing and Communications, pp. 1520-1524. Gao, M., Zhang, Q., Ni, L., Liu, Y. and Tang, X. (2012), Cardiosentinal: A 24-hour heart care and monitoring system, Journal of Computing Science and Engineering, 6(1), 67-78.

Goh, E.J. (2003), Secure indexes, IACR Cryptol. ePrint Arch., p.216.

Goh, E.J.(2001), Secure indexes, IACR Cryptol. ePrint Arch., p.216-217.

Goh, E.J., Shacham, H., Modadugu, N. and Boneh, D. (2003), SiRiUS: Securing Remote Untrusted Storage. NDSS, 3(2), 131-145. Gong, T., Huang, H., Li, P., Zhang, K. and Jiang, H. (2015), A medical healthcare system for privacy protection based on IoT in Seventh International Symposium on Parallel Architectures, Algorithms and Programming (PAAP), IEEE, pp. 217-222.

Goyal, V., Pandey, O., Sahai, A. and Waters, B. (2006), Attribute-based encryption for fine-grained access control of encrypted data, in Proceedings of the 13th ACM conference on Computer and communications security, pp. 89-98.

Green, J. (2014), The Internet of Things Reference Model, In the Internet of Things World Forum, pp. 1-12.

Groce, A. and Katz, J. (2010), A new framework for efficient password-based authenticated key exchange, in Proceedings of the 17th ACM conference on Computer and communications Security, pp. 516-525.

Groce, A. and Katz, J. (2010), A new framework for efficient password-based authenticated key exchange, in Proceedings of the 17th ACM conference on Computer and communications security, pp. 516-525.

Groce, A. and Katz, J. (2010), October. A new framework for efficient password-based authenticated key exchange, in Proceedings of the 17th ACM Conference on Computer and Communications Security , pp. 516-525.

Grnbk, I. (2008), Architecture for the Internet of Things (IoT): API and interconnect, in Second International Conference on Sensor Technologies and Applications (sensor-comm 2008), pp. 802-807.

Hammi, M.T., Livolant, E., Bellot, P., Serhrouchni, A. and Minet, P. (2017), A Lightweight Mutual Authentication Protocol for the IoT, in Proceedings of International Conference on Mobile and Wireless Technology, pp. 3-12.

Hassan, M.M., Lin, K., Yue, X. and Wan, J. (2017), A Multimedia healthcare data sharing approach through cloud-based body area Network, Future Generation Computer Systems, 66(4) , 48-58.

Hassanalieragh, M., Page, A., Soyata, T., Sharma, G., Aktas, M., Mateos, G., Kantarci, Healthcare: from IoT to Cloud Computing, SCIENTIA SINICA Informations, 43(4), 515-528.

Hedi, I., peh, I. and arabok, A. (2017), IoT network protocols comparison for the purpose of IoT constrained networks ,in 40th International Convention on Information and Communication Technology, Electronics and Microelectronics (MIPRO),IEEE, pp. 501-505.

Hong, N. (2013), A security framework for the internet of things based on public key infrastructure, Advanced Materials Research,67(2),3223-3226.

Hu, J.X., Chen, C.L., Fan, C.L. and Wang, K.H. (2017), An intelligent and secure health monitoring scheme using IoT sensor based on cloud computing, Journal of Sensors.

Huang, M., Liu, A., Wang, T. and Huang, C. (2018),Green data gathering under delaydifferentiated services constraint for Internet of Things, Wireless Communications andMobileComputing.

Hwang, J.J. and Yeh, T.C. (2002), Improvement on Peyravian-Zunic's password authentication schemes, IEICE Transactions on Communications, 85(4), pp.823-825.

Imadali, S., Karanasiou, A., Petrescu, A., Sifniadis, I., Vque, V. and Angelidis, P. (2012), eHealth service support in IPv6 vehicular networks, in IEEE 8th International Conference on Wireless and Mobile Computing, Networking and Communications (WiMob), pp. 579-585.

Issariyakul, T. and Hossain, E. (2009), Introduction to network simulator 2 (NS2), Introduction to network simulator NS2, Springer, Boston, MA, pp. 1-18.

Istepanian, R.S. (2011), The potential of Internet of Things (IoT) for assisted living applications, in IET Seminar on Assisted Living 2011, pp. 1-40

Istepanian, R.S., Hu, S., Philip, N.Y. and Sungoor, A. (2011), The potential of the Internet of m-health Things m-IoT for non-invasive glucose level sensing in Annual International Conference of the IEEE Engineering in Medicine and Biology Society , pp. 5264-5266.

Istepanian, R.S., Hu, S., Philip, N.Y. and Sungoor, A. (2011), The potential of Internet of m-health Things M-IoT for non-invasive glucose level sensing, in Proceedings of Annual International Conference of the IEEE Engineering in Medicine and Biology Society, pp. 5264-5266.

Istepanian, R.S., Jovanov, E. and Zhang, Y.T. (2004), Guest editorial introduction to the special section on m-health: Beyond seamless mobility and global wireless healthcare connectivity, IEEE Transactions on Information Technology in biomedicine, 8(4), 405-414.

Jara, A.J., Alcolea, A.F., Zamora, M.A., Skarmeta, A.G. and Alsaedy, M.(2010), Drugs interaction checker based on IoT, Internet of Things (IoT), 6(2), 1-8.

Jian, Z., Zhanli, W. and Zhuang, M. (2012), Temperature measurement system and method based on home gateway, Chinese Patent, 102811185.

Jiang, Q., Lian, X., Yang, C., Ma, J., Tian, Y. and Yang, Y.(2016), A bilinear pairing based anonymous authentication scheme in wireless body area networks for mHealth., Journal of Medical Systems, 40(11), 231- 232.

Jing, Q., Vasilakos, A.V., Wan, J., Lu, J. and Qiu, D. (2014), Security of the Internet of Things: perspectives and challenges, Wireless Networks, 20(8), 2481-2501.

Kallahalla, M., Riedel, E., Swaminathan, R., Wang, Q. and Fu, K. (2003), Plutus: Scalable Secure File Sharing on Untrusted Storage,. Paper presented at 2nd USENIX Conference on File and Storage Technologies, FAST 2003, San Francisco, United States.In Fast 3, 29-42.

Kang, M., Park, E., Cho, B.H. and Lee, K.S. (2018), Recent patient health monitoring platforms incorporating Internet of Things enabled Smart Devices, International Neurourology Journal, 22(Suppl 2), p.S76.

Khemissa, H. and Tandjaoui, D. (2015), A Lightweight Authentication Scheme for E-health applications in the context of Internet of Things, in 9th InternationalConference on Next Generation Mobile Applications, Services and Technologies IEEE, pp. 90-95.

Kinkelin, H., Hauner, V., Niedermayer, H. and Carle, G. (2018), Trustworthy configuration management for networked devices using distributed ledgers, in NOMS 2018-2018 IEEE/IFIP Network Operations and Management Symposium, pp. 1-5.

Kothmayr, T., Schmitt, C., Hu, W., Brnig, M. and Carle, G. (2012), A DTLS based end-to-end security architecture for the Internet of Things with two-way authentication, in Proceedings of 37th Annual IEEE Conference on Local Computer Networks-Workshops, pp. 956-963.

Kothmayr, T., Schmitt, C., Hu, W., Brnig, M. and Carle, G. (2013), DTLS based security and two-way authentication for the Internet of Things, Ad Hoc Networks, 11(8), 2710-2723.

Kouicem, D.E., Bouabdallah, A. and Lakhlef, H(2018), Internet of Things security: A top-down survey, Computer Networks, 141(2), 199-221.

Krasnova, A (2017). Smart invaders of private matters: Privacy of communication on the Internet and in the Internet of Things (IoT). PhD thesis. Radboud University
Lamport, L. (1981), Password authentication with insecure Communication, Communications of the ACM, 24(11), 770-772.
Laranjo, I., Macedo, J. and Santos, A. (2013), Internet of Things for medicationcontrol: E-health architecture and service implementation, International Journal ofReliableand QualityE-Healthcare (IJRQEH), 2(3),1-15.

Lee, J.Y., Lin, W.C. and Huang, Y.H. (2014), A lightweight authentication protocol for Internet of Things, in International Symposium on Next-Generation Electronics (ISNE),

IEEE, pp. 1-2.

Li, C.T., Lee, C.C. and Weng, C.Y. (2016), A secure cloud-assisted wireless body area network in mobile emergency medical care system, Journal of Medical Systems, 40(5), 117-117.

Li, J., Chen, X., Li, M., Li, J., Lee, P.P. and Lou, W. (2013), Secure deduplication with efficient and reliable convergent key management, IEEE Transactions on Parallel and Distributed Systems, 25(6), 1615-1625.

Li, M., Yu, S., Cao, N. and Lou, W. (2011), Authorized private keyword search over encrypted data in cloud computing, in 31st International Conference on Distributed Computing Systems IEEE, pp. 383-392.

Li, M., Yu, S., Zheng, Y., Ren, K. and Lou, W. (2012), Scalable and secure sharing of personal health records in cloud computing using attribute-based encryption, IEEE transactions on parallel and distributed systems, 24(1), 131-143.

Lionel, M.N., ZHANG, Q., TAN, H., LUO, W. and TANG, X.(2013), Smart Liu, D., Ning, P. and Li, R. (2005), Establishing Pairwise Keys in Distributed SensorNetworks, ACM Transactions on Information and System Security (TISSEC), 8(1),41-77.

Liu, F. and Li, T. (2018), A clustering-anonymity privacy-preserving method for wearable IoT devices, Security and Communication Networks, 20(1), 112-116.

Liu, M.L., Tao, L. and Yan, Z. (2012), Internet of Things-based electrocardiogram monitoring system, Chinese Patent, 102(7),118.

Lounis, A., Hadjidj, A., Bouabdallah, A. and Challal, Y. (2013), Secure medical architecture on the cloud using wireless sensor networks for emergency management. in Eighth International Conference on Broadband and Wireless Computing, Communication and Applications, IEEE, pp. 248-252.

Lounis, A., Hadjidj, A., Bouabdallah, A. and Challal, Y. (2016), Healing on the cloud: Secure cloud architecture for medical wireless sensor networks, Future Generation Computer Systems, 55(4), 266-277.

Ma, Y., Zhang, Y., Wan, J., Zhang, D. and Pan, N. (2015), Robot and cloud-assisted multi-modal healthcare system. Cluster Computing, 18(3), 1295-1306.

Machaka, P., Bagula, A. and Nelwamondo, F. (2016), Using exponentially weighted moving average algorithm to defend against DDoS attacks, in Pattern Recognition Association of South Africa and Robotics and Mechatronics International Conference (PRASA-RobMech) IEEE, pp. 1-6.

Mahmoud, R., Yousuf, T., Aloul, F. and Zualkernan, I. (2015), Internet of Things (IoT) security: Current status, challenges and prospective measures. in 10th International Conference for Internet Technology and Secured Transactions (ICITST), pp. 336-341.

Manyika, J., Chui, M., Bisson, P., Woetzel, J., Dobbs, R., Bughin, J. and Aharon, D. (2015), Unlocking the Potential of the Internet of Things, McKinsey Global Institute, 20 (4), 40-47.

Medaglia, C.M. and Serbanati, A. (2010), An overview of privacy and security issues in the Internet of Things, The internet of things, 65(12), 389-395.

Medaglia, C.M. and Serbanati, A. (2010), An overview of privacy and security issues in the internet of things, The Internet of Things Springer, New York, NY, pp. 389-395.

Medaglia, C.M.,and Serbanati, A. (2010). An Overview of Privacy and Security Issues in the Internet of Things, The Internet of Things, Springer, New York, NY, pp. 389- 395.

Miao, Y., Ma, J., Liu, X., Wei, F., Liu, Z. and Wang, X.A. (2016), m 2-ABKS: Mishra, D., Srinivas, J. and Mukhopadhyay, S. (2014.), A secure and efficient chaotic map-based authenticated key agreement scheme for telecare medicine information systems, Journal of Medical Systems, 38(10), 120-120.

Moghaddam, F.F., Moghaddam, S.G., Rouzbeh, S., Araghi, S.K., Alibeigi, N.M. and Varnosfaderani, S.D. (2014), A scalable and efficient user authentication scheme for cloud computing environments, in 2014 IEEE Region 10 Symposium , pp. 508-513.

Mohammed, N., Fung, B.C., Hung, P.C. and Lee, C.K. (2010), Centralized and distributed anonymization for high-dimensional healthcare data, ACM Transactions on Knowledge Discovery from Data (TKDD), 4(4), 1-33.

Mosa, A.S.M., Yoo, I. and Sheets, L. (2012), A systematic review of healthcare applications for smartphones, BMC medical informatics and decision making, 12(1), 67-67.

Mukherjee, A. (2015), Physical-layer security in the Internet of Things: Sensing and communication confidentiality under resource constraint, in Proceedings of the IEEE, 103(10), pp.1747-1761.

Murillo-Escobar, M.A., Cardoza-Avendao, L., Lpez-Gutirrez, R.M. and Cruz- Hernndez, C. (2017), A double chaotic layer encryption algorithm for clinical signals in telemedicine. Journal of Medical Systems, 41(4), 59-59.

Na, S., Hwang, D., Shin, W. and Kim, K.H. (2017), Scenario and counter measure for replay attack using join request messages in LoRaWAN, in Proceedings of International Conference on Information Networking (ICOIN) IEEE, pp. 718-720.

Nastase, L. (2017), Security in the internet of things: A survey on application layer protocols, in 2017 21st International Conference on Control Systems and Computer Science (CSCS), IEEE, pp. 659-666.

Nijmegen.

Ning, H.S. and Xu, Q.Y. (2010), Research on global Internet of Things' developments and its construction in Chi,.Dianzi Xuebao(Acta Electronica Sinica), 38(11), 2590-2599.

Ouaddah, A., Mousannif, H., Abou Elkalam, A. and Ouahman, A.A. (2017), Access control in the Internet of Things: Big challenges and new opportunities, Computer Networks, 112 (4), 237-262.

Palattella, M.R., Accettura, N., Vilajosana, X., Watteyne, T., Grieco, L.A., Boggia, G. and Dohler, M. (2012), Standardized protocol stack for the internet of (important) things, IEEE communications surveys and tutorials, 15(3), 1389-1406.

Pammu, A.A., Chong, K.S., Ho, W.G. and Gwee, B.H. (2016), Interceptive side channel attack on AES-128 wireless communications for IoT applications, in IEEE Asia Pacific Conference on Circuits and Systems (APCCAS), pp. 650-653.

Pang, Z., Tian, J. and Chen, Q. (2014), Intelligent packaging and intelligent medicine box for medication management towards the Internet-of-Things, in IEEE International Conference on Advanced Communication Technology , pp. 352-360.

Pascu, T., White, M., Beloff, N., Patoli, Z. and Barker, L. (2013), Ambient health monitoring: The smartphone as a body sensor network component, InImpact: The Journal of Innovation Impact, 6(1), 62-65.

Pilkington, M. (2017), Can Blockchain improve healthcare management? Consumer medical electronics and the IoMT, Consumer Medical Electronics and the IoMT.

Porambage, P., Schmitt, C., Kumar, P., Gurtov, A. and Ylianttila, M. (2014), Two-phase authentication protocol for wireless sensor networks in distributed IoT applications, in IEEE Wireless Communications and Networking Conference (WCNC), pp. 2728-2733.

Pranata, H., Athauda, R. and Skinner, G. (2012), Securing and governing access in ad-hoc networks of Internet of Things, in Proceedings of the IASTED International Conference on Engineering and Applied Science, EAS, pp. 84-90.

Puustjrvi, J. and Puustjrvi, L. (2011), Automating remote monitoring and information therapy: An opportunity to practice telemedicine in developing countries, in IEEE 2011 IST-Africa Conference Proceedings , pp. 1-9.

Rahmani, A.M., Gia, T.N., Negash, B., Anzanpour, A., Azimi, I., Jiang, M. and Liljeberg, P. (2018), Exploiting Smart e-Health gateways at the edge of Healthcare Internet-of-Things: A fog Computing Approach, Future Generation Computer Systems, 78 (2), 641-658.

Raju, D.N. and Saritha, V. (2016), Architecture for fault tolerance in mobile cloud computing using disease resistance approach, International Journal of Communication Networks and Information Security, 8(2), 112.

Raju, D.N. and Saritha, V. (2016), Architecture for fault tolerance in mobile cloud computing using disease resistance approach, International Journal of Communication Networks and Information Security, 8(2), 112-114.

Raju, D.N. and Saritha, V. (2018), A Survey on Communication Issues in Mobile Cloud Computing, Walailak Journal of Science and Technology (WJST), 15(1), 1-17.

Ruiz, M.N., Garca, J.M. and Fernndez, B.M. (2009), Body temperature and its importance as a vital constant, Revista de enfermeria (Barcelona, Spain), 32(9), 44- 52.

Scarpato, N., Pieroni, A., Di Nunzio, L. and Fallucchi, F. (2017), E-health-IoT universe: A review, International Journal on Advanced Science Engineering Information

Technology, 7(6), 4467.

Schmitt, C., Noack, M. and Stiller, B. (2016), TinyTO: Two-way authentication for constrained devices in the Internet of Things, In Internet of Things, 40(5), 239-258.

Shahamabadi, M.S., Ali, B.B.M., Varahram, P. and Jara, A.J. (2013), A network mobility solution based on 6LoWPAN hospital wireless sensor network (NEMO- HWSN), in Seventh International Conference on Innovative Mobile and Internet Services in Ubiquitous Computing , pp. 433-438.

Shahamabadi, M.S., Ali, B.B.M., Varahram, P. and Jara, A.J. (2013), A network mobility solution based on 6LoWPAN hospital wireless sensor network (NEMO- HWSN), in Proceedings of Seventh International Conference on Innovative Mobile and Internet Services in Ubiquitous Computing IEEE, pp. 433-438.

Sharma, S. and Sharma, S.(2016), A defensive timestamp approach to detect and mitigate the Sybil attack in vanet, in Proceedings of 2nd International Conference on Contemporary Computing and Informatics (IC3I) , IEEE, pp. 386-38.

Shen, J., Gui, Z., Ji, S., Shen, J., Tan, H. and Tang, Y. (2018), Cloud-aided lightweight certificateless authentication protocol with anonymity for wireless body area Networks. Journal of Network and Computer Applications, 106,117-123.

Singh, D., Tripathi, G. and Jara, A.J. (2014), A survey of Internet-of-Things: Future vision, architecture, challenges, and services, in IEEE world forum on Internet of Things (WF-IoT), pp. 287-292.

Singh, R., Singh, J. and Singh, R. (2016), Cluster Head Authentication Technique against Hello Flood Attack in Wireless Sensor Networks, International Journal of Computer Applications, 156, 43-49.

Sinha, S., Singh, A., Gupta, R. and Singh, S. (2018), Authentication and tamper detection in tele-medicine using zero watermarking, Procedia computer science, 132, 557-562.

Song, C., Lin, X., Shen, X. and Luo, H. (2013), Kernel regression based encrypted images compression for e-healthcare systems, in International Conference on Wireless Communications and Signal Processing, IEEE, pp. 1-6.

Song, D.X., Wagner, D. and Perrig, A. (2000), Practical techniques for searches on encrypted data, in Proceeding of IEEE Symposium on Security and Privacy. SandP 2000, pp. 44-55.

Song, D.X., Wagner, D. and Perrig, A. (2000), Practical techniques for searches on encrypted data, in Proceeding 2000 IEEE Symposium on Security and Privacy. SandP 2000 IEEE, pp. 44-55.

Song, Z., Zhang, Y. and Wu, C. (2011), A reliable transmission scheme for security and protection system based on internet of things, in Proceedings of the IET International Conference on Communication Technology and Application (ICCTA 11), pp. 806810.

Swiatek, P. and Rucinski, A. (2013), IoT as a service system for eHealth. in IEEE 15th International Conference on e-Health Networking, Applications and Services (Healthcom 2013), pp. 81-84.

Thota, C., Sundarasekar, R., Manogaran, G., Varatharajan, R. and Priyan, M.K. (2018), Centralized fog computing security platform for IoT and cloud in healthcare system, Fog computing: Breakthroughs in research and practice,10(4), 365-378.

Trnka, M., Cerny, T. and Stickney, N. (2018), Survey of Authentication and Authorization for the Internet of Things, Security and Communication Networks, 10(7), 1-14.

Tschofenig, H., Arkko, J., Thaler, D. and McPherson, D. (2015), Architectural Considerations in Smart Object Networking, RFC 7452, 1-24.

Tseng, F.H., Chou, L.D. and Chao, H.C. (2011), A survey of black hole attacks in wireless mobile ad hoc networks, Human-centric Computing and Information Sciences, 1(1), 4.

Turkanovic, M., Brumen, B. and Hlbl, M. (2014), A novel user authentication and key agreement scheme for heterogeneous ad hoc wireless sensor networks, based on the Internet of Things notion, Ad Hoc Networks, 20(4), 96-112.

Uher, J., Mennecke, R.G. and Farroha, B.S. (2016), Denial of Sleep attacks in Bluetooth Low Energy wireless sensor networks, in MILCOM 2016-2016 IEEE Military Communications Conference IEEE,pp. 1231-1236.

Vazquez-Briseno, M., Navarro-Cota, C., Nieto-Hipolito, J.I., Jimenez-Garcia, E. and

Sanchez-Lopez, J.D. (2012), A proposal for using the internet of things concept to increase children's health awareness, in CONIELECOMP 2012, 22nd International Conference on Electrical Communications and Computers, pp. 168-172. IEEE.

Venkatesh, V. and Parthasarathi, P. (2013), Trusted third party auditing to improve the cloud storage security, Wireless Communication, 5(4), pp. 183-187.

Viswanathan, E. K. Lee, and D. Pompili. (2012), Mobile grid computing for data- and patient-centric ubiquitous healthcare, in Proceedings. 1st IEEE Workshop Enabling Technol. Smartphone Internet of Things (ETSIoT), pp. 36-41.

Wan, J., Zou, C., Ullah, S., Lai, C.F., Zhou, M. and Wang, X. (2013), Cloud-enabled wireless body area networks for pervasive healthcare, IEEE Network, 27(5), 56-61.

Wang, B., Zhang, H., Wang, Z. and Wang, Y. (2008), A secure mutual password authentication scheme with user anonymity, Geomatics and Information Science of Wuhan University, 33(10), 1073-1075.

Wang, F., Hu, L., Zhou, J. and Zhao, K. (2015), A data processing middleware based on SOA for the Internet of Things., Journal of Sensors, 15 (2), 43-49.

Weyrich, M. and Ebert, C. (2015), Reference architectures for the Internet of Things, IEEE Software, 33(1), 12-15.

Whitmore, A., Agarwal, A. and Da Xu, L. (2015), The Internet of ThingsA survey of topics and trends, Information systems frontiers, 17(2), 261-274.

Wu, Z.Q., Zhou, Y.W. and Ma, J.F. (2011), A security Transmission Model for Internet of Things, Jisuanji Xuebao (Chinese Journal of Computers), 34(8), 1351-1364.

Wu, Z.Q., Zhou, Y.W. and Ma, J.F. (2011), A security transmission model for internet of things, Jisuanji Xuebao (Chinese Journal of Computers), 34(8), 1351-1364.

Wu, Z.Q., Zhou, Y.W. and Ma, J.F. (2011), A security transmission model for Internet of Things, Jisuanji Xuebao (Chinese Journal of Computers), 34(8), 1351-1364.

Wu, Z.Y., Lee, Y.C., Lai, F., Lee, H.C. and Chung, Y. (2012), A secure authentication scheme for telecare medicine information systems, Journal of Medical Systems, 36(3), 1529-1535.

Xiao, Y., Chen, X., Li, W., Liu, B. and Fang, D. (2013), An immune theory based health monitoring and risk evaluation of earthen sites with Internet of Things in International Conference on Green Computing and Communications and IEEE Internet of Things and IEEE Cyber, Physical and Social Computing, pp. 378-382.

Xiaopeng, G. and Wei, C. (2007), A novel gray hole attack detection scheme for mobile ad-hoc Networks, in IFIP International Conference on Network and Parallel Computing Workshops (NPC 2007) , pp. 209-214.

Xie, W.J. (2013), A Secure Communication Scheme Based on Multipath Transportation for the Internet of Things, South China University of Technology, Guangzhou, China, 37(9), 135-142.

Yang, H., Kim, H. and Mtonga, K. (2015), An efficient privacy-preserving authentication scheme with adaptive key evolution in remote health monitoring system, Peer-to-Peer Networking and Applications, 8(6), 1059-1069.

Yang, J.J., Li, J.Q. and Niu, Y. (2015), A hybrid solution for privacy preserving medical data sharing in the cloud environment, Future Generation computer systems, 43(4), 74-86.

Yang, K., Forte, D. and Tehrani poor, M.M. (2015), Protecting endpoint devices in IoT supply chain, in IEEE/ACM International Conference on Computer-Aided Design (ICCAD), pp. 351-356.

Yang, L., Ge, Y., Li, W., Rao, W. and Shen, W. (2014), A home mobile healthcare system for wheelchair users in Proceedings of the 2014 IEEE 18th international Conference on Computer Supported Cooperative Work in Design (CSCWD), pp. 609- 614.

Yang, N., Zhao, X. and Zhang, H. (2012), A Non-contact health monitoring model based on the Internet of Things, in8th International Conference on Natural Computation, pp. 506-510.

Yang, Y. (2015), Attribute-based data retrieval with semantic keyword search for e-health Cloud. Journal of Cloud Computing, 4(1), 10-11.

Yao, X., Chen, Z. and Tian, Y. (2015), A lightweight attribute-based encryption scheme for the Internet of Things, Future Generation Computer Systems, 49(4), 104- 112.

Ye, N., Zhu, Y., Wang, R.C., Malekian, R. and Lin, Q.M. (2014), An efficient authentication and access control scheme for perception layer of the Internet of Things, ACM Transactions on Information and System Security (TISSEC), 12(2), 229- 248.

You, L., Liu, C. and Tong, S. (2011), Community medical network (CMN): Architecture and implementation in IEEE Global Mobile Congress , pp. 1-6.

Zhang, J., Chen, D., Zhao, J., He, M., Wang, Y. and Zhang, Q. (2012), Rass: A portable real-time automatic sleep scoring system, in IEEE 33rd Real-Time Systems Symposium, pp. 105-114.

Zhang, K., Liang, X., Lu, R. and Shen, X. (2014), Sybil attacks and their defenses in the Internet of Things, IEEE Internet of Things Journal, 1(5), 372-383.

Zhang, X.M. and Zhang, N. (2011), An open, secure and flexible platform based on Internet of Things and cloud computing for ambient aiding living and telemedicine, in International Conference on Computer and Management (CAMAN), pp. 1-4.

Zhang, Y., Chen, M., Huang, D., Wu, D. and Li, Y. (2017), iDoctor: Personalized and professionalized medical recommendations based on hybrid matrix factorization, Future Generation Computer Systems, 66 (8), 30-35.

Zhao, W., Wang, C. and Nakahira, Y. (2011), Medical application on Internet of Things, in Proceedings IET International Conference on Communication Technology Applications (ICCTA), pp. 660-665.

Zhao, Y. (2016), Identity-concealed authenticated encryption and key exchange in Proceedings of the 2016 ACM SIGSAC Conference on Computer and Communications Security, pp. 1464-147.

Zhao, Y.L. (2013), Research on data security technology in the internet of thing, Applied Mechanics and Materials, Trans Tech Publications Ltd, 433, 1752- 1755.

Zheng, X.H., Chen, N., Chen, Z., Rong, C.M., Chen, G.L. and Guo, W.Z. (2014), Mobile cloud based framework for remote-resident Multimedia Discovery and Access,Journal of Internet Techmnology, 15(6), pp.1043-1050.

Zhenhua, D., Jintao, L. and Bo, F. (2009), Research on hash-based RFID security authentication protocol, Journal of Computer Research and Development, 46(4), 583- 584.

Zhenhua, D., Jintao, L. and Bo, F. (2009), Research on hash-based RFID security authentication protocol, Journal of Computer Research and Development, 46(4), 583- 585.

Zhou, Jun et al. (2017). Security and privacy for cloud-based IoT: challenges. In: IEEE Communications Magazine 55.1, pp. 2633.

Zhu, B., Addada, V.G.K., Setia, S., Jajodia, S. and Roy, S. (2007), Efficient distributed detection of node replication attacks in sensor networks, in Twenty- Third Annual Computer Security Applications Conference (ACSAC 2007) IEEE, pp. 257-267.

Zhu,Q.,Wang,R.,Chen,Q.,Liu,Y.andQin,W.(2010),IoT gateway:Bridgingwireless sensor networks into the Internet of Things, inIEEE/IFIP InternationalConference on Embedded andUbiquitous Computing, pp.347-352.

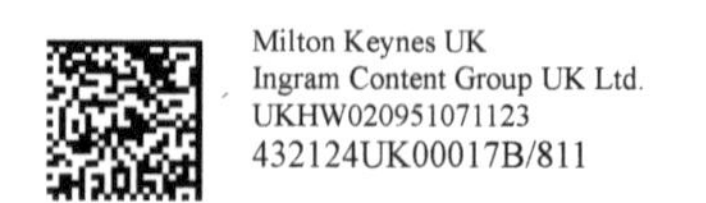
Milton Keynes UK
Ingram Content Group UK Ltd.
UKHW020951071123
432124UK00017B/811